# My Heart Transplant For Your Amusement

**Vince Clews**

Copyright © 2020 by Vince Clews
All Rights Reserved
ISBN9798606326402

This book is dedicated to
Carol Clews.

"When she walked into the room,
it became home."
Thank you, Lord, for this woman.

There is no way to express the faithfulness of her visits and the joy they brought without a special acknowledgment to my daughter, Ashleigh Clews.

# Table of Contents

Letter to Donor Family ................................................. ix

Acknowledgments ...................................................... xi

Introduction .............................................................. xvii

1. *Le Moribund* ......................................................... 1

2. Bad News from Reggio di Calabria .................. 14

3. Johns (that's with an "s") Hopkins ................... 20

4. Accepted…Maybe .............................................. 27

5. 2.1 and Counting ................................................ 35

6. The Woman Who Did Not Lie ......................... 42

7. The Man on the Platform .................................. 47

8. ♪Party Pooper, Party Pooper♪ ........................... 51

9. The Other Side of the Mat ................................. 58

10. It Ain't Dancing, But It'll Do ........................... 67

11. An Aging Pachyderm in an Open Gown ........ 78

12. Carol, the Warden ............................................ 84

13. The Best Piece of Advice Ever ....................... 93

14. No Rest for the Weary .................................... 102

15. Right Where I Needed to Be .......................... 107

16. A New York Kind of Girl.................113

17. Get Naked.................121

18. A Lesson About Birds.................127

19. Exactly Right.................135

20. Chopped Beef Patties Are Flat.................148

21. A Day at the Races.................156

22. Sepsis, Sepsis.................159

23. Up My Nose with a Ten-Foot Hose.................166

24. THE Call.................176

25. Joy in the Morning.................183

26. Alive and Aware . . . Well, Alive.................188

27. Back on My Feet?.................202

28. Christmas, Too?.................208

29. "If You Can Wait and Not Be Tired by Waiting"*
.................213

30. Passing Homes Lit for Christmas.................220

Postscript.................226

Appendix.................230

About the Author.................259

# Letter to the Donor Family

On March 3, 2015, I sent the following letter to the donor family via The Living Legacy Foundation of Maryland.*

My name is Vince Clews. On October 27, 2013, I became the beneficiary of a heart transplant. I can only write this note to you today because of the selfless, generous, and courageous act of your family. I am a writer and, still, I am unable to express in words what your donation has meant to me and to those around me who were also beneficiaries of your decision. I suspect that you donated multiple organs on behalf of your son. That, of course, means that there are multiple families who daily thank God for you and your strength.

I am so sorry for your loss. I know that no amount of thanks from his recipients can ever provide consolation equal to your grief. Please know that the world your son's life will affect is greater than you can ever imagine. The ripple effect that results from that one touch of his soul on the water of time is a blessing that will continue to have an impact on lives far wider, and for far longer, than you will ever be blessed to know. I can tell you that with the certainty of a recipient. Lives will be changed forever, the lives of his recipients and those individuals they will touch who will then touch others. That is God's gift to you ... His absolute message that the life with whom He entrusted you, for even just a short time, will live far beyond a meager life's expectancy.

I pray that He will bless you with "the peace that passes all understanding" and that you will be given strength in the knowledge you have been God's good and faithful servant.

*I later learned that the letter I wrote minus, of course, my name was received by the family and that they had declined to respond. I completely understand. Apparently, this is not unusual. For now, they know they have my everlasting appreciation and love. I encourage each recipient to write to his or her donor family.

# Acknowledgments

*So much goes into doing a transplant operation. All the way from preparing the patient to procuring the donor. It is like being an astronaut. The astronaut gets all the way to the moon, but he had nothing to do with the creation of the rocket or navigating the ship. He's the privileged one who gets to drive to the moon.*
—Dr. Denton Cooley
The first American doctor to perform
a heart transplant, on May 3, 1968

These acknowledgments have to begin by recognizing the people who most deserve it. They are the members of the family of the young man whose heart lives on in me. There is nothing I can ever do to appropriately thank them.

This might also be the appropriate time to acknowledge the groundbreaking donor and recipient for their significant roles in heart transplantation. Denise Darvell was the person whose heart was donated so that another life could be saved. Louis Washkansky was the recipient. He lived only eighteen days. But they opened the cardiac transplant door that, forty-six years later, I entered.

I am indebted to so many people that I will surely leave out some I should include. If you are reading this and your name is not here and you know it should be, I apologize. The ordeal and creeping age have tempered my memory, but not my gratitude. I thank all those who helped make the transplant process tolerable, successful, and, at times, amusing. You will find many of their names throughout the book.

How do people survive a difficult ordeal without strong family support? I am glad I do not know the answer to that question. I have, without a doubt, the best family in the world. Not just my immediate family, but also my extended family. You will meet many of them through this book. I wish you could do it in person. You would love them, too. I want to especially acknowledge my late parents. They are now in heaven with special mansions. God's way of saying "I'm sorry" for having stuck them with me.

My thanks to Dr. James Porterfield, who first diagnosed the source and extent of my heart problems, as well as to Dr. Stuart Russell, who initiated my stay on the Johns Hopkins Hospital cardiac transplant list. And thank you to the entire cardiac transplant team at the University of Maryland Medical Center (UMMC), where my heart transplant was finally performed.

My very special thanks to Dr. Erika D. Feller, Founder and Medical Director of the University of Maryland Cardiac Transplant Program. Dr. Feller is also my cardiologist. I, and every member of my family and my friends, cannot thank her enough for saving my life. From moment one, she gave my family and me every reason to believe I would live. I also extend my gratitude to her staff who was, and continues to be, a perfect extension of her expertise and care. I write often of Dr. Feller throughout this book. As you learn more about her, you will understand why I treasure her as a physician and delight in my time with her.

To Drs. Si M. Pham and Keshava Rajagopal, the surgeons who worked overtime to transplant a vibrant heart for a dying one, thank you. And thanks to those who assisted in the operating room through the long hours of my surgery. You kept me alive and assured my good health.

I have to say a special thanks to the cardiac care nurses at UMMC who not only gave me expert medical attention but also made life worth living during a six-month hospital stay. You are angels on earth. I love you all.

And thank you to the "techs"—the people who made sure that both I and my bed were clean and that my personal needs were met. They brought light, kindness, humor, and loving care into my room all day and night long.

Thanks to the housekeeping staff. They did a thankless task with such attention and care that you would have thought they had high-paying jobs. Amazing.

During my stays, both at the hospital and at the Kernan Rehabilitation Center, the work of the rehabilitation staff whose members got me back on my feet and walking again is surely appreciated, as is that of those folks who continued to help me when I got home.

I have a circle of wonderful friends despite the fact that I should not. They were kind and helpful from my first signs of weakness through my full recovery. I especially want to thank them for the way they were always there for not only me, but also for Carol. One friend made sure she had an escort to the many activities and events Carol's job required she attend. I want to thank him for being gay.

Because my dad was a minister, I have known clergy throughout my life. Some have had a very positive influence on me. Perhaps none so much as the late Rev. Philip Burwell Roulette. He was my minister when my illness was diagnosed. He retired before my transplant but made certain to visit regularly and each time to give me a blessing before he left. He was my dear friend.

My minister as I grew increasingly ill, and at the time of my transplant, was Rev. David Drake. David is a prayer warrior. His prayers for my strength and healing empowered me. His prayers for, and attention to, Carol helped both of us find comfort and the peace of the Lord during times of doubt and fear.

My thanks to the prayer warriors who held me up for everything from faith issues to healing—from family to friends through fellow congregants at Church of the Resurrection (Lutherville, Maryland). Of note there was Vic Meyer, whose booming "Voice of God" prayers raised the beams every Sunday from first sign of my illness to complete recovery. To people I never knew and still do not, I cannot adequately express the feeling of serenity I had knowing I was being lifted up by someone somewhere almost around the clock. And my sister, Marcia, who will lead prayer meetings in heaven, made sure of that.

There would be no *My Heart Transplant for Your Amusement* had not Ashleigh created a CarePages site that she and Carol maintained from my diagnosis through my homecoming. Family and friends were able to access the site, get regular updates, and enter messages of love and encouragement ... mostly love, always encouragement. If you ever have a family member who is ill or in a hospital for any length of time, I urge you to set up a site for messages to the patient. We used CarePages which, I am disappointed to say, no longer exists. CarePages provided a free online scrapbook of sorts where friends and family members could read about my progress and also leave encouraging notes for me. What a wonderful repository of hope and love my pages were. As I wrote this book, I referred to that site for information I did not know or simply would have forgotten. You may be able to find a similar site currently active on the Internet. Please find it and use it. And send cards. Plenty of cards.

During the course of writing and rewriting this book, it has been edited at various stages by Libbye Morris, Dedi Whitaker, Fran Minakowski, and Amy Nugent. I thank each one for bearing with me and my inability to stop making errors and changes. Amy, showing extreme patience with me, edited the version you are reading and prepared it for publication.

The cover design for the book was created by Stephen Wiley. Steve is the eldest son of my dearest friend for over fifty years, the late Tom Wiley. Steve offered to create the cover as a tribute to, and in memory of, his artist father and his mother, Mary.

This acknowledgment would be incomplete if I did not note the work of the United Network for

Organ Sharing (UNOS) and other organ-donor, recipient, and coordinating organizations. *Be a donor*.

I know this series of acknowledgments has been lengthy. Hopefully, you will never find out how hard it is to shorten the list of people you want to thank who were instrumental in saving your life.

Finally, to you, thank you for your interest in my retrospective ramblings.

# Introduction

I can write this book only because I have been the beneficiary of a family so filled with grace that it made the decision, even in its moments of deepest grief, to allow me—and, I feel certain, other beneficiaries—to live when life was slipping away. What an example of extraordinary selflessness, of love for people you do not even know. I want to again send a message to members of that family. *In reference to the title and tone of the book, I find nothing humorous about the loss of your loved one nor the grief you are experiencing.* I can assure you that there is not one single sentence in this book that treats your loss, or the life, of your young relative lightly or with any humor.

So why, then, *My Heart Transplant for Your Amusement*? Simply, my mind tends to see humor in what others think "isn't so damn funny." Even when I was in the hospital, and sometimes in some pretty bad pain, I found moments of humor. It is the way a mind like mine works. Let me see if I can help make it clear by using artists and paintings. With apologies to comparing my mind to his, think of Picasso and his paintings. When people who write humor see the world it just does not look like what other people see. That is the best I can do to explain it.

My wife, Carol, who suffered through incredibly difficult times with me and stayed strong for me, was not always amused by the circumstances. Nor were my children, brother, sister, and other members of my extended family. I do not blame them. Honestly, without question, this whole episode was far harder on them than on me. But they have all lived with me long enough to expect this treatment of my heart transplant. In fact, now and again, they laughed with me.

I should call attention to the extensive dialogue in this book. Very little of it is verbatim. In fact, and especially in the humorous exchanges, it is doubtful that we talked with punch lines at the ends of our sentences. But the dialogue does indicate the nature of the exchanges we had. Where medical people were speaking, I generally tried to reflect the situation, not their exact words.

Once again, I want to emphasize that the title and tone of this book might seem disrespectful of the donor process. Not at all, not ever.

I want this book to bring to prospective organ recipients a greater sense of relaxation about the often daunting process of waiting for, and then recovering from, a heart transplant. The good news is that the wait is the hardest part. The time period from the transplant surgery to release from the hospital is normally a matter of weeks. The trials and tribulations I went through during my transplant process are the exception. That is why I can write a book about it. So, my fellow heart transplant patients-to-be, forge ahead without fear, despite what I have written.

I hope each of you will be encouraged to make the same generous decision my donor family did. The person whose life you save, and extend, will find great joy in the additional years … and so may you.

Finally, and again, if you are not already, *be a donor*.

# Chapter 1
## *Le Moribund*

*If you did not read the Acknowledgments and the Introduction, I urge you to go back and read them before you continue.*

I grew up a healthy kid, maturing—and I use that word loosely—into an equally healthy, physically active adult. With one exception. All that time, I was unknowingly carrying a fatal disease just waiting to launch its deadly attack.

I was born in Richmond, Virginia, in 1943, shortly before Yankees were no longer known as Carpetbaggers. At least not all of them. Apparently, the doctor who delivered me found no evidence of the disease in my system. There is no record of it. Well, there may have been, but the hospital burned down in 1994, and with that, many of its records were lost.

I spent most of my early career as a writer/producer for public television and the subsequent years freelancing those same talents. In my early fifties, I was hired to produce a video for a faith-based organization and its worldwide food distribution and development programs. The assignment required traveling for six weeks to developing countries. Most of those regions were in hot climates: Central America, Africa, the Mideast, and Southeast Asia. Lots of mountainous and rugged terrain, even a couple of deserts. There were times when I was tired, but fifty years is, after all, half a century old.

Ten years later, I was hired to do the same kind of traveling for another organization, this one focused on conflict resolution. I returned to Southeast Asia, Africa, and, this time, I also spent some time in the mountains of Macedonia, Kosovo, and Albania. When we began the trip, I was in good physical shape, actually comfortable in my clothes—a big barometer for me. Once again, we were very active. My food consumption was moderate. However, as we moved from location to location, my clothes got increasingly uncomfortable. I recall being in the back of an open jeep in Africa, sitting on some of our equipment cases, wondering how in the heck a pair of formerly loose jeans and an oversized sweatshirt got so tight. The answer could have been better.

My wife, Carol, was the first to sense that there was a serious problem. It occurred one night when we were going to a banquet. I dropped her off at the door and found a parking spot close by, maybe ten or fifteen yards away, up a short incline to the door. As I began the walk toward Carol, I suddenly realized that my legs were weak and I was out of breath. "Out of breath" was not even in my vocabulary. I played a lot of tennis. I could play three successive matches without needing a break. That did not mean I won all of them. But I was there. I also was a runner. I could run several miles and not be really winded when I finished. Okay, that was when I was younger, before I had to have both knees replaced. However, I had remained in pretty good shape, and I could still work hard in the yard on a hot, humid day and not be exhausted. I was blessed with stamina.

However, on the night of the banquet, things were different. When I got to Carol, I was breathing like a fat penguin looking into the open mouth of an Orca whale. Although I was unaware of it then, my chances of survival were not much better than the penguin's. Carol blurted out, "What's wrong with you?" I had no answer. Even if I had, I would have had to wait until I got my breath to deliver it. Carol was ready to call an ambulance, but I dismissed the incident. In a short time, I was breathing normally. I noted that I had no pain in my chest, or in my arm, or any place else that I did not normally have pain. I reminded her that we were not spring chickens. Sometimes I feel like I never learn. In spite of my ignorance, an otherwise pleasant evening was often interrupted by Carol asking me, "How do you feel? Are you okay?" I was feeling fine, and I told her so—a reassurance always followed by Carol adding, "I don't believe you." The truth is that I did feel fine. So I moved on from the episode. Until the next day.

The next day was Sunday. We got up, got dressed, and went to church. I dropped Carol off at the front door and drove down a short incline to the parking lot. As I was walking up the hill, I realized I was breathing hard. I had walked this route every Sunday, and some weeks more often than that. I had never become winded. "Well, that's it. No more seconds." I had a tendency to put on weight, and I had noticed that getting to the regular notch on my belt was requiring that little extra pull. I had never been uncomfortably fat. Maybe that is only because

I had worked at keeping my weight somewhere between "Well, he's not obese" and "He could afford to lose a few pounds."

I could get pretty serious about the weight matter, too. I once ate only canned sardines and yogurt for weeks. That was back when yogurt had the consistency of liquid plastic. And tasted like it, too. During that experiment, I did not have a lot of problems with people invading my breathing space. That was then. But now I was struggling to walk up the hill to church. When I reached the front door, I was breathing pretty hard. A couple of the greeters by the front door asked me if I was all right. I was sort of asking myself the same thing.

It did not matter where I went—if there was an incline, when I got to the top I had to take a moment to catch my breath. I continued to attribute the problem to the weight I obviously was gaining. So I addressed the issue as I always had: I cut back on my eating. That was always well before Thanksgiving. After that, and through the New Year, well, normally I treated that period as if I were a bear needing to prepare for winter hibernation. I have always been particularly fond of Thanksgiving season. I see the color of the autumn leaves as spectacular and am in awe of their beauty. And they have a certain aroma. One part the fresh air rushing through them, and the other is the musk that comes with moldering. Where I live it becomes cold as fall unfolds, and every smell seems to separate and become more intense. At least for me, that is so. Of course, I have a rather enlarged proboscis. It can take in much more air than the average person.

*LE MORIBUND*

As fall advanced into winter, I seemed to have hit new goals in my hibernation prep. Carol, who has always reminded me that she prefers a man with a little bit of a belly, apparently decided I was taking the concept beyond her fancy. Actually, she was concerned that I had begun having increased problems breathing at progressively lesser inclines. Our mailbox is a short walk down the driveway. No problem getting there. Bringing the mail back to the house, however, was leaving me increasingly out of breath. I often would stay outside until I got my breath and then walk inside so Carol would not know I was struggling. The flaw in the plan was that by the time I got inside I was breathing hard again. Finally, Carol had had it. She insisted that we see our family doctor. Note something now. It is the word "we." Remember that.

The doctor's appointment was brief. He shared Carol's concern and connected us with a cardiologist. An appointment was made, and on that date we showed up. Carol wanted us to take the stairs to his third-floor office so the doctor could witness my gasping for breath. I did not see the point of walking up the two flights just to make me breathe hard. I suggested we could achieve the same result by taking the elevator and making out hard with a lot of hands-on time. We took the steps. By the time we reached the second floor, I was already breathing hard. Climbing the next flight was even worse. We walked into the doctor's office with me in full breathless mode. After we sat reading out-of-date magazines for twenty minutes, I was breathing perfectly fine.

We had a couple of subsequent appointments with the doctor, whose interests were varied and did not include me. Each session concluded with Carol saying, "Can we talk about my husband's heart?" On our way out after the third appointment, I stopped to schedule the next one. Carol said, too loudly as far as I was concerned, "Never mind, we're not coming back here," and marched out with me following, apologizing to everyone. I still will not go to that floor in the medical building for fear of seeing someone from that office. But she was right.

The decision, of course, left us without a cardiologist. I decided to die writing at my desk, which is in our home. To add drama to the event, I got out the very old typewriter I first used when I began my writing career. I moved my computer and put the aged Underwood on my desk. The scene was very theatrical. I sat down and began to type. Carol shrugged off my idiosyncratic behavior. She had more important things to do…like finding a new cardiologist. And she found one.

My first impression was that Dr. Porterfield looked like the kindly doctor in the old movies and TV shows from my childhood. That was comforting. As soon as the doctor listened to my irregular heartbeat, he laid out what was going on. I was in atrial fibrillation (a-fib). The American Medical Association describes a-fib as "a quivering or irregular heartbeat (arrhythmia) that can lead to blood clots, stroke, heart failure, and other heart-related complications." I might add here that if you look up *arrhythmia* at other places on the internet, the definition often adds, "possibly resulting in death." I would call that a "heart-related complication." The doctor suggested that I lose twenty pounds. "Twenty pounds?!" I could not see myself giving up all those foods it would take to drop that much weight. I love food. Actually, it is eating I love. Sitting around the table with family and a bunch of friends eating a heaping bowl of spaghetti, talking, eating some more, never letting the conversation lapse. Eating until the bowl is empty, staying at the table talking, enjoying antipasti, and emptying bottles of wine. To me, eating is a celebration of life. *Mangia, mangia.*

I lost not only the twenty pounds the doctor wanted me to lose, I lost a whole thirty. That was because we did not "Vince eat." We "Carol ate." She reminded me often, "You're going to do what the doctor said." Three months later and thirty pounds less, you would have thought I would have been swimming in my clothes. Wrong. I was still belly too big. Clearly concerned, the doc ordered an abdominal scan. From that scan he determined that the weight was not fat. Rather, it was fluid in my abdominal tissue. I thought, "Okay. I can sweat that out." I had just seen some sort of plastic exercise suit they were selling on TV. The user runs in it to help lose water weight. "I'll get one of those and wear it all the time. Even when I write. Problem solved." I can see life so simply. During one of our (note the plural) succeeding sessions with Dr. Porterfield, he informed us that fluid problems sometimes have more serious ramifications than a little water in the belly. He shared that sometimes excess fluid could be related to possible heart issues. Carol must have asked what was done in situations like that, and the doctor said it would depend on the seriousness of the problem. In the gamut of treatment measures the doctor may have mentioned, at the extreme, a heart transplant. Frankly, it went right past me. But Carol heard it. And it stuck. If extreme measures had to be taken to save her husband, then that is what *we* would do.

Carol watched closely as I increasingly struggled to find the energy to perform even the easiest of physical tasks. Like sleeping. During the night, I would wake up gasping for air. My gasps often came out like screams, where the air went inward instead of out. The gasps were loud. They scared the crap out of me. In addition to the horror show I was putting on, I would be awakened with Charlie horses in my lower legs, particularly the left one. Holy Mother of God, did they hurt. At first, I would try to stay in bed and stretch them out. No luck. I soon found out that I needed to get up and walk. I would walk up and down the hall, into rooms, around them, and back out into the hall. Up and down, again and again. It would usually take between five and ten minutes to relieve the pain. These episodes would frequent my sleep several times a night. They were very disruptive for both of us.

So, let's see. We were going to awaken for the day at 5:00 a.m. Carol was then going to shower, get dressed, drive about an hour-plus in heavy traffic, then work until 5:00 p.m., drive an hour-plus back home in more traffic and, because she insisted, make dinner for us. We would go to bed around 10:00 p.m., get up at 5:00 a.m. and begin the cycle again. And there I was, her bedmate, waking several times a night, loudly gasping for air, kicking my legs around, and getting up and walking around the house like some sort of nocturnal creature out of a vintage B&W horror film. I suggested that I move to the guest room and sleep there. Carol would have none of that. "What if you're in trouble and I don't know it?" Fat chance of that. There was a graveyard near our home. Even the corpses were asking where all the commotion was coming from.

Carol researched my symptoms, and the more she read, the more often the words "heart transplant" came up. When Ernie, my brother-in-law who, due to his work, knew a great deal about medicine affirmed her suspicions, she became intent that we find out more about the transplant option. As she gathered information, she was increasingly encouraged. Every time the transplant procedure came up in discussion, she would say things like, "Thank God, we have an answer to our prayers." Let me see if I got this right. We were talking about cutting me open from my Adam's apple to my ass. Oh, yeah, that was sure an answer to my prayers.

I was still so certain the problem was fat that I was not seriously concerned about any kind of surgical possibility, let alone a heart transplant. Carol wanted me alive, no matter what it took. So she hung onto those two words "heart transplant" like a terrier with a bone. She talked with people about it like we had won an all-expenses-paid Roman holiday cruise. I saw it as a rowboat ride across the river Styx. One of the friends Carol shared her great news with was a nurse supervisor at the world-renowned Johns

Hopkins Hospital (JHH) located right in our hometown, Baltimore, Maryland. The friend arranged for me (I am sorry, us) to meet with an influential doctor associated with the hospital. You do not turn down an invitation to see a doctor at Hopkins. That just is not done in proper circles. So a meeting was arranged. After only one visit, he put us in touch with a Hopkins cardiologist. It took the doctor no time to concur that my heart was in arrhythmia. The first attempt to fix my problem was electro-cardioversion. The purpose was to shock my heart back into rhythm. At first, it worked. I felt great. However, the a-fib quickly returned. He tried again. Once again, it took but did not hold. Now we were in deeper waters.

The problem was congestive heart failure. But not routine congestive heart failure. Not me. Tests indicated that my situation was caused by amyloidosis. I should probably define that word right now. Internet site WebMD.com has this to say about it: "Amyloidosis is a condition in which an abnormal protein called amyloid builds up in your tissues and organs. When it does, it affects their shape and how they work. Amyloidosis is a serious health problem that can lead to life-threatening organ failure." Life-threatening organ failure. And I had that in my heart? Yes, that sounded "life-threatening" to me. One other note about the disease. There is no cure for amyloidosis.

We met with the new doctor to discuss where we go from here. He was young and forthright. I do not remember his exact words, but to Carol's ears they came out, "Mr. Clews is going to die." I could feel her immediate reaction in the chair next to me. Her jaw tightened. I could not tell if she was fighting back tears or furious that the doctor had been that forthright. It turned out that she was trying not to cry. At first. Then her defensive mechanism set in. She resented being told something that uncompromising about her husband's fate and was not buying it. I do not know if she heard the doctor talking about options for treating the problem. I sure did not. I was completely focused on Carol's jaw getting tighter and tighter. She did not loosen it until we were well away from the doctor's office. In the name of decency, I really cannot write what she said after we were down the hall and around the corner. Carol never went to another appointment with him. She could not deal with a doctor she heard say I was going to die. I tried to remind her that he was merely the messenger. Nope. Not going back. I was not going to die. She held on to that pledge from that day forward. It was a pledge written on the bone held tight in her jaw. And she was not going to let go.

Carol has a much stronger faith than I have. She diligently studies the Bible, when on good days, I only tend to blow the dust off mine. She prays every day for herself and people she loves, knows, even those she does not know, and, most remarkably, those she does not love. My attempts at prayer must leave God turning to Gabriel and saying, "Well, that's just downright embarrassing." Her faith is a train. Mine is a train set. Yet she had a terribly difficult time accepting the situation. At times she was flat-out angry with God and told Him so. Frankly, I did not see where that was helpful.

Generally, when she gets angry with someone, she can be pretty tough on that person and, in turn, that person gets pretty angry back. I just did not see this as a good time to create any ill will with God toward our household. I was in enough trouble as it was.

There was a tough moment for us during a church service one Sunday. Several months prior, I had been asked to read the New Testament passage for that week. The passage was from Revelation 24:4. In spite of the projections of a better time, it was hard for me to read and for Carol to hear. "And God shall wipe away all tears from their eyes, and there shall be no more death, neither sorrow, nor crying, neither shall there be any more pain; for the former things are passed away." I got through it. Carol listening, just barely. The poor fellow who much earlier, well before my prognosis, assigned me that reading could not apologize enough. If he could have "rent his clothes" and "heaped ashes on his head," he could not have been more apologetic. I felt sorrier for him than I did for myself.

I continued to meet with the doctor, always making an excuse for Carol's absence. It turns out she did not miss many appointments. The doctor soon accepted a job at another hospital and was gone. The next doctor saw me for a few weeks, and then he, too, accepted a job elsewhere and moved away. Two doctors, both getting the hell out of Dodge ASAP after meeting with me. With Hopkins losing docs at that rate, I expected to get a letter from the front office: "Dear Mr. Clews. You must find another hospital," and signed with a signature I could not read.

*LE MORIBUND*

It turned out that Hopkins did not give up so easily. The new ball carrier was an all-star. He was the chair of the cardiac transplant committee at the hospital, Dr. Stuart Russell. Dr. Russell, meet Carol. Carol, show the doctor your bone.

# Chapter 2
# Bad News from Reggio di Calabria

Dr. Russell knew all about heart transplantation and soon all about me. And, very quickly about Carol and Terrier grip.

He acted promptly to move the process forward. He scheduled follow-up tests. The results led to a meeting with a panel of Hopkins staff members. I cannot remember what all of them did, but I am sure there were doctors in the group. I later had the suspicion some psychiatrists were there. Probably lawyers and bean counters, too. I also thought there was some concern about the reason for my amyloidosis.

It seems there are two main causes for the disease. One was, at that time, called *senile amyloidosis*. In that case, the person is seventy-five or older. I was sixty-nine at the time. So that eliminated me from senile amyloidosis. What an unkind name. Frankly, I was glad I was not part of that group. And, thank you anyhow, I would just as soon not be invited to join. The other group was those who had familial, or *hereditary, amyloidosis*. Now we were into an area of possibility. I was told there are pockets of the world where people are more prone to get the disease. One is a small port city in southern Italy, Reggio di Calabria. And guess what?

That was where my mother was born. So I may have gotten it from my mom. If she wanted to perpetuate the memory of my Italian genes, I'd have happily settled for Pavarotti's voice.

Guess who did not get the amyloid gene? My brother, Carter. Of course not. Mommy's favorite. I am not kidding. It was a family joke my brother particularly enjoys. I once found a picture of a mother bird feeding a worm to her two babies. Actually, to one of them. As she stood at the nest, dangling the worm to one of the hatchlings, one foot was on the nest and the second one was firmly planted on the head of the other hatchling. Our whole family agreed it was a picture of mom, Carter, and me. Enough of Carter. Back to me. Oh, wait, my sister did not get amyloidosis, either. Marcia was clean. I suspect that if it was in her system, her good, Christian living flushed it out before it hurt her. In other words, God was on her side, too. In Marcia's case, well deserved.

In order to know more, the study team drew blood samples and sent bloodwork to a lab in Boston that they were certain would confirm the Italian connection. The results came back. *No!* (You have to say it with Italian emphasis). The Hopkins team, certain there was an error, had blood drawn again and sent it to the Boston group to test once more. Even the crew up there thought they must have made a mistake the first time. Nope. No trace of Reggio. And remember, the only other type of amyloidosis was the senile form, a term I am pleased to note they no longer use. I am, as far as I know to this day, an anomaly. I am the one who has amyloidosis who got it for no explicable reason. I am not so sure I would be gloating if I had died. Actually, I am not so sure I am gloating now.

While all this was going on, I was continuing to have an increasingly difficult time getting around. The fluid buildup in my tissue was manifesting itself in my very noticeable weight gain. In simple terms, I was fluid fat. Nonetheless, fat. Side-show "Fat Man" fat. Talk about depressing. And debilitating. I could hardly get from my big old recliner to the bathroom to urinate. And when I did make it, my groin area was so bloated with fluid from the illness and my penis so withdrawn into the bloat that I nearly peed all over myself before I could get a grip. I am here to tell you, bloat and recalcitrance is not a pretty picture. The doctor put me on diuretics. At first, they worked. I peed a lot and was holding my own. Ha, I just realized what I wrote. I am keeping it. As for peeing, you can pee only so much. My weakened heart was losing its battle, and my body was joining the retreat. All in all, I was very sick. My appearance and my limited mobility reminded me of that every moment.

Bolder action was required. So I was assigned to the Johns Hopkins Heart Failure Bridge Clinic. Interesting name. I was immediately reminded of a bridge I once had to cross that may have helped account for my heart failure. It was in Freetown, the capital of Sierra Leone. At that time, my production company was there to document a group of people who led desperately poor lives. They lived in an open area beneath the city where some buildings had fallen and were never restored. The only way to get to their embankment dwelling area was to cross a "bridge" over a polluted stream. The bridge was a fifty-something-foot strip of wood that looked like an undersized railroad tie. During my travels as a video producer, I have been in a few life-threatening situations, but I have never been so certain I was going to die as I was if I fell in that dirty stream. I was looking down at water that had, I feel fairly certain, as yet undiscovered disease-carrying microbes. When we got across the rail, we had to walk along the stream on muddy, slippery banks. Shoe manufacturers are decades away from the sole design that would hold on that slime. The people living there washed their clothes in that stream and, possibly, drank from it. They called their community Bone Suffer. Bone Suffer, surely because the residents suffered to the bone. The name was written in paint on a big slab from a fallen building. I was better off dying from heart disease than those people were just living.

When I went to my introductory session at the Heart Failure Bridge Clinic, Carol, of course, joined me. We were escorted to a room with a desk and several recliners, where we were greeted by friendly nurses. Their job was, essentially, to cause me to pee. A lot. I would visit once a week, and they would shoot me up with diuretics to open the floodgates. And, boy, did it work. I would spend several hours—sometimes four or five—there while I made trips back and forth to the toilet, where I would pee voluminous, hard-rushing streams. I mean, like a horse. Holy cow, did it work. One day I dropped seven pounds. When the frequency of the toilet trips on a given visit would slow, I would go home.

The fluid release worked. The walk through a tunnel from the parking lot to their pee-atorium was especially long. When I began my visits, I was carrying so much fluid in my bloated body that I could barely complete the walk. I was always exhausted and breathing very hard when I arrived at the clinic. But I showed up for every session. On time. For a guy who spent his life saying, "Nobody tells me what to do," I folded like a cheap accordion for these people. Call me Compliant Clews. The sessions worked. By the sixth week, I was Fred Astair-ing through the tunnel. I was lighter than I had been in months. Then, boom!—they stopped the treatments. Although I was losing fluid, the process was pounding my kidneys. It took just a few weeks after the treatments stopped for me to put all the weight back on. All retained fluid. This phenomenon was generally apparent in my midsection. Very unattractive. And my damaged heart was getting worse. I thought we should do something about the way I looked with a disproportionate belly. Carol and the doctors were more concerned about my heart. Where was their sense of pride in appearance?

Someone told me at one point, and I do not know who this was, that the bloating was a part of what the exit stages would be like. So I figured I was at the beginning of the end. It came so quickly. I began to quietly go about preparing for it as much as I could. I called the local funeral home to find out how cremation was handled. I wanted to meet with them alone to make arrangements. Asking Carol to go seemed like rubbing hot coals into an open wound. I began to plan my funeral service. And I started a final letter to be read at the service: "First, I want to thank all of you for being here today. I'm sure you would rather be doing something else. Just for the record, so would I."

It was on the tail end of my "pee 'til you drop visits" that Carol met with Dr. Russell. I was there, too. As the session appeared to be drawing to a close, he shared the news. The transplant team at the hospital had talked informally about me and my situation. They believed I might be a good candidate for a heart transplant. Carol's eyes welled up, and she muttered, "Thank you, Lord." What's with the "Thank you, Lord"? The doctor just suggested cutting a gaping hole in my chest? But, in reality, I had been presented with an incredible opportunity—an opportunity to live beyond my current life span. During Carol's celebratory moment, I had a startling thought: "Oh, my God, I'm going to outlive my term life insurance."

# Chapter 3
# Johns (that's with an "s") Hopkins

Based on Dr. Russell's news, we thought we had better start getting ready for a pending hospital stay. But the doctor did not call, and he did not write. He did not even email. Carol became very concerned and, at times, a bit angry. The longer we waited, the more her jaw tightened around that bone.

I was more relaxed about the wait. At least I thought I was. One day I was at my desk writing when I heard the nearby repeated roar of a motorcycle on the road in front of the house. On top of making that abhorrent noise, every once in a while the cyclist would stop to rev the engine right where it was most disruptive. He also used the same spot to "pop wheelies." I finally had had enough. I walked outside and strolled to the edge of the road. I waited for him. As he approached, I waved him down. He stopped. When he removed his helmet, I spoke.

"I just wanted to ask you to keep doing those high-speed wheelies."

He looked at me like I was nuts.

"I'm waiting for a heart transplant. You look like you have the kind of young, healthy heart I need. If you kill yourself right here in front of my house, it would wildly increase my chances to get my transplant now."

The rider studied me as if he did not understand what I said. He probably did not. Anyone who would carry on the way he was could not be too smart. He put his helmet back on and sped away, perhaps to kill himself, dammit, in front of someone else's home. Yeah, I guess I was feeling the stress.

Finally, after about six weeks, we got a call from Tracey, the administrator for the transplant team. She wanted to talk about schedules so they could begin creating a time period for the interviews and tests that were to follow to determine if the transplant process was going to move forward. If she could, Tracey said, she would schedule the tests and procedures during a two-day period. That was nice of her. Johns Hopkins was not that far away from our home, but it is on the other side of the city, and it takes a while to get there.

At the meeting, one of the first things we were told was that the interviewers like the spouse of the prospective recipient to be involved throughout the process. "You just hit the mother lode," I said, but wisely, under my breath. The coordinator set up an additional series of meetings and tests. At the first one, we were presented with all the ins and outs of the assessment process that would help determine "if you make the list."

"*If?* I'm dying here, lady."

"People who are 1A, who are very sick, are at the top of the list."

Okay, that's me.

"The next group down is the 1Bs. Then there are the 2s, a 2B being at the very bottom of the list. You will go on the list as a 2B."

Then this little tripwire from one of the people in the room: "I've been doing this job for over nineteen years, and I've never seen a 2B get a heart."

I could feel the wind come out of Carol's sails. Mine went a little flaccid, too.

Another of the early meetings was with a group of doctors to talk about my circumstances and for them to present information regarding a transplant. Most of it was routine—as routine as you can get when you are talking about a heart transplant. I recall only one moment. I caught everyone off-guard, including Carol. "I've decided that I should pass on this surgery."

There was a forty-week pregnant pause. My reasoning, as I explained, was that I was sixty-nine years old and I had lived a good life.

"I was blessed to be raised in a good home with loving parents. I have terrific siblings. I have a wonderful wife and children who love me. My career was spent doing exactly what I wanted to do. I have been healthy, until now. I know where I'm going when I die. In other words, life has been good to me. I think the heart I would get should go to a younger man so he can experience the joy in life I have known. And so that he can be with his wife for added years and live to raise his children."

I said it, and I meant it. There was a poignant beat. Then one of the doctors calmly explained that there was no reason to take a pass on a heart. He said the one I would get would be such a perfect fit for me that there was no guarantee that, at the moment it would be available, there would be another recipient so specifically suited for it. I am still not sure if they thought I was noble or nuts. I know what Carol thought because the whole ride home she told me, in no uncertain terms.

Throughout the series of meetings, my favorites were the ones with the social worker, Helen, an energetic woman of whom I initially was very suspicious. She began the first session by noting the stress that can build during the wait for a matching heart. It can be difficult on everyone in the family. She wanted to know how patient we saw ourselves during stressful times. Carol began to answer, but Helen interrupted her: "What's the story on this guy's fuse?"

Carol noted that, on small matters, I have little patience, but that on major issues, I seem to be about as patient as anyone she has ever known. The social worker saw that as a positive. I said, off-handedly, "Carol has no patience with anything." The social worker dismissed my comment as nonsense, later noting that in the short time she had spent with us, she had already come to the conclusion that Carol must be a woman of great patience. Carol and she became instant best friends. Then Helen followed up on her anger question.

"Is he prone to violent outbursts, like putting his fist through a wall?"

Carol said she had never seen me get physical.

"I used to hit walls, but I grew up when I married Carol, and now I only hit people."

I did not really say that, but it went through my mind as a very funny comeback. I let discretion be the better part of funny and just smiled like the town idiot. I have a confession to make here. There was a piece of information I decided Helen did not need to know. My maternal grandfather, Vincent Marciano, was a self-reliant Italian who immigrated to this country in the early 1900s. He was a tough little man who was patently unpleasant. When he was in his late nineties, he was in a nursing home. Apparently his roommate was a screamer, especially at night. After unsuccessfully asking that either he or the man be moved to another room, one night, Granddad got up and beat the man to death. Yeah, she does not need to know that. Not now.

The social worker was very thorough, and Carol listened carefully. I was beginning to get tired and just wanted to go home and take a nap. Finally, she asked if we thought all the members of the family were going to be supportive.

Carol told her, "Vince, his siblings, and all the kids are like the Mafia about 'family first'." Helen said she would like to meet again, next time with the whole family. Carol said she would work on setting it up. I asked if I had to be there, as I had heard it all before. No one laughed. Wasted humor.

The second meeting with Helen came together nicely. It was set for a date when my son, Chris, was going to be visiting from his Florida home. The entire immediate family was there, including our friend, Michael, who is one of the family, rather like the gay brother I never had. He was introduced only as a dear friend; his lifestyle choice has never been an issue.

Helen brought up many of the matters we had discussed at the earlier meeting to gauge the collective opinions. I hasten to add, she was still interested in the subject of my anger. "Come on, Helen, for God's sake. Move on, or I'm going to turn over this damn table." Another one of those things I thought would have been funny to say, but I knew better than to say it. It turned out that I did not need to provide the humor. Helen did it, without even knowing, with another anger question: "Let's take an example. How do you think Mr. Clews would react if, say, Mrs. Clews ran off with your friend Michael?"

There was a pregnant pause, and then Chris answered, "With utter shock."

There was laughter around the table except for poor Helen, who must have wondered what was so funny. When we told her that Michael was gay, she laughed harder than any of us. That was our last meeting with Helen. We enjoyed her company so much that I considered throwing a chair through a window just to see her again.

On a more serious note, the issue of my kidneys had been overshadowed by the focus on my dying heart. But it was not forgotten. I met with the nephrologist. An aside: During this incident, I happened to be listening to a series of recordings on the history of the pharaohs. There was an entire lesson on Queen Nefertiti. At one point during our first meeting I imagined the nephrologist wearing the Queen's cap crown. *Nephrology. Nefertiti.* I know. Very immature. If you have not figured out that about me by now, you have not been reading carefully.

WebMD.com explains my specific kidney problem this way: "The diminished volume of blood pumped out by the heart (decreased cardiac output) is responsible for a decreased flow of blood to the kidneys. As a result, the kidneys sense that there is a reduction of the blood volume in the body. To counter the seeming loss of fluid, the kidneys retain salt and water. In this instance, the kidneys are fooled into thinking that the body needs to retain more fluid volume when, in fact, the body already is holding too much fluid."

So that was why I was holding water and looking fat. It was not the Italian subs after all.

The last appointment that day was for carotid testing. It was painless and over without issue. Everything for the day was completed, and we were finally on our way to the car. I was exhausted and could barely make the walk to the garage. Carol drove home, and I slept. On those occasions when I have seen a woman driving and a man sleeping in the passenger seat, I have always assumed, as I bet most of us do, the guy is drunk or lazy. I was so passed out for the ride home that I am sure people thought, "Pretty early for the guy to be that drunk. Poor woman. What she must put up with." I now know that the guy in the passenger seat could not give a hoot what we think.

What a day.

# Chapter 4
# Accepted…Maybe

We once had a great dog named Sam. Sam went to work with me every day. My office was an old house on Main Street, about a mile and a half from our home. One morning, when I called Sam to leave, he did not respond. We called and called. Nothing. Finally, we decided to search for him. We live on a country road, but it sometimes has heavy traffic in the mornings. If you have a dog, you know the sick feeling you get when you think it may have been hit by a car and is lying somewhere in pain. We searched and searched, up and down the road, looking in gullies and checking every side street. No Sam. Finally, I told Carol I had to get to the office and left the search to her.

When I arrived at the office, there was Sam, patiently waiting for me to open the door. I was told later that all the rides back and forth had left just enough scent for him to be able to get there on his own. In the following weeks and months we, or sometimes I (can you believe it?), went to Hopkins for tests and meetings so many times that eventually, I got into the car, backed out of the garage, sat back, and let the car follow its fumes to the hospital.

I am not medically savvy enough to recall all the tests I was given during that time, but I do remember two.

## MY HEART TRANSPLANT FOR YOUR AMUSEMENT

The first test I recall was a computerized tomography scan (CT scan, or cat scan). There were two problems here. First, I did not like to lie on my back. I never have. That was especially so during my illness when I was having trouble breathing. I was laid on my back on a sliding table that was pushed into a tiny tube. Second, I have claustrophobia. "Small spaces" and the name "Vince Clews" should never be in the same sentence. Did I say the CT was scheduled for Friday the 13th? Friday the 13th. In spite of all my concerns, there I was. Once I was in the tube, a small tube, I was cautioned not to move. I was in this small tube, I could not breathe, and…I need to stop for a…I can't breathe. And, while I was in this small…I need to step outside for a moment. Excuse me. I'll …

Okay, I am back. Needless to say, the cat scan was not a great experience.

The second procedure of the day was a heart biopsy. Lying on my back again. The process involved running a tube into the artery on the right side of my neck and shoving it into my heart. The tube had a pincher that took a microscopic bit of the organ for the test. I was hoping the result would be that they discovered a soon-to-be-written world-class piece of writing that had not yet found its way to my pen. All they unearthed was disease. Just my luck.

The doctors were doing these tests for two reasons. The cat scan was to see if my lungs were strong enough to sustain me through the surgery and recovery. They were. The second reason was to see if my heart was really as bad as the reports had indicated. It was. And perhaps worse. A lot worse. I thought, "Fine. They're going to reject me. I can go home." But to the doctor, the results were good news. What? How can it be good that I am closer to dying? He told us that it helped bump me up on the list of those waiting for a heart—to 1A, possibly. That sounded like good news, I guess. If you have to be on the list at all.

The findings were reported to a group called "the transplant team." They could approve proceeding or send me packing. We were told when they would be meeting. We were also told that they usually met early in the morning. Tracey was to let us know what they decided. Carol and I waited by the phone. Hour after hour. No call. At four o'clock, I decided that this was one of those situations like applying for a job. They call you all happy if you got it. If you did not, they send you a letter. I envisioned the letter being something brief and to the point: "Dear Mr. Clews. Make sure your estate is in order." And then signed with a signature I could not read. Boy, Carol was going to be devastated.

Shortly after four o'clock, the phone rang. It was the call.

"Mr. Clews, I'm so excited to tell you the team has tentatively accepted you for a heart transplant."

I turned to Carol. "I'm in, but...."

Carol did not hear the "but." She began to cry.

"Oh, God. Thank you, Lord."

It was a special feeling to see my wife cry tears of joy after having seen so many tears of anguish. Of course, there was that word, "tentatively." My damaged kidneys were still in the mix. The doctors needed to run more tests. The cardiac surgeons had had conversations with the nephrologists and, together, had come to a tentative conclusion that a new heart would, in large part, resolve my still-existing kidney problems. That would mean dodging a simultaneous heart/kidney transplant. Still, they needed to be certain. And, frankly, they needed to reassure some doubters that I should even have the surgery.

So there was another test. They ran a different kind of catheter from my neck into my heart. Then they performed magic and gave my heart a normal rhythm. They looked at how the kidneys responded to a healthier heart. As with almost everything in life, there was a little X factor. If the test showed the kidneys were not healing, the team of doctors would wash their hands of the whole thing. Well, at least that was my impression. If, on the other hand, the kidneys showed signs of recovery, I would stay on the transplant list. I needed only one kidney to show adequate strength. That is because we can live with only one functioning kidney. Two is better. But one is good enough.

The test indicated that my kidneys would respond. I was going to be admitted to Johns Hopkins Hospital for a heart/kidney transplant with the full expectation that the latter would not be necessary. We were scheduled to tour the ward where I would wait for my new heart. In fairness, that line should read, "…where *we* would wait for my new heart." Every hour I would spend in that room was an hour that Carol also spent waiting, wherever she was.

Because I was now a patient waiting for admittance, we were scheduled for more regular meetings. The logical parking lot for us to use was the one nearest the cardiac care unit. There is an especially long walkway from the garage to the building. Now, I do not get how an organization that spends millions of dollars on a building where heart patients are treated does not put a moving walkway from the garage to the entrance. Forget the "Oh, the walk is good exercise for heart patients" excuse. If you have heart problems, that walk is not good exercise; it is a Bataan Death March.

We were met by Tracey, the young woman who had been with us during most of our previous meetings and had made the good-news call. She was going to give us a tour. My daughter, Ashleigh, joined us. It was a sign of the interest, concern, and compassion she would continue to display for the remainder of my journey. I think the deal may also have been that she would report back to the other siblings. We headed toward the intensive care unit. Carol fell behind. She had stepped into a little cove in the hall. Reality had hit again. She was crying. It was such a difficult moment. I wanted to go to her and hold her, but I could see she was trying to act as if she was looking at something on the wall. I finally walked over and put my arm around her. We all waited while she composed herself. At that moment, she seemed so vulnerable, and I felt utterly distressed for her. What was I doing to her? She had been pretty strong through all of this, but there were moments for both of us when it felt like we had walked over hot coals into a wall, and it had knocked us right back

## MY HEART TRANSPLANT FOR YOUR AMUSEMENT

into the ashes. This was obviously one of those moments for her. Being the strong woman she is, she pulled herself together and apologized. We pointed out that that was unnecessary, and we continued to the ward.

The tour was, at once, fascinating, startling, and...well, now that I think about it, startling. I must tell you that because it was "the" Hopkins, I thought I was going to have a suite. You know, like a Marriott. Close your eyes for a moment and picture one. Yeah, that is what I saw. We proceeded into the ward and into reality. First, we could see into all the rooms. The wall facing the hall was glass. What kind of privacy is that? Then we walked into an unoccupied room. The first item I saw was a bed with an uncomfortable-looking mattress. Then a vinyl chair and couch. I did see a TV screen. Overall, however, it was pretty sparse. On scanning the room further, I noticed that I did not see a door for a bathroom.

"Where's the bathroom?"

Tracey walked over to a thing that looked like a free-standing commode.

"Here."

"That's it?"

"That's it, on rare occasions when you can leave your bed. You're going to be pretty confined to your bed and monitored twenty-four hours a day. There can't be anything that blocks their view. You understand, don't you?"

A nod was the best I could muster. Suddenly this was looking pretty bleak.

## ACCEPTED... MAYBE

When I was in high school, I did not always stay on the path my parents set for me. Stay on the path? How about shooting off to another planet? The local high school did not work out so well for me. At the end of my freshman year, there was not a lot of teacher enthusiasm for my return. Let's just say it: I was a bad student and a worse kid. My father thought I needed a more disciplined, but faith-based, academic situation away from the comfort of home life. He found such a school, just over two-thousand miles away in western Canada. Mother, surprisingly, would hear none of that. It was one of those St. George and the Dragon moments we children often got to observe during our growing years. Dad's compromise with my distressed mother was a mere fifteen hundred miles away in South Carolina. I spent my sophomore high school year there. On Sunday afternoons, each academy student was compelled to join one of the college student groups to go on day-mission trips. One of my roommates invited me to join his group, which I did. This was 1958. The school was in the Deep South—1958 Deep South. My group went to the camps where the chain gangs were "housed." A better word might be "cooped." Remember the movie *Cool Hand Luke*? They nailed it. Coops. That is what the prisoners lived in. "Chicken coops" with beds running along the outside walls. As I recall, each prisoner was ankle-cuffed to a chain that was locked to his bed. The chain was just long enough to allow him to get to one of a series of barrels that lined the middle of the coop. Those barrels were their toilets.

# MY HEART TRANSPLANT FOR YOUR AMUSEMENT

It seemed to me at the moment in the hospital tour, when my prospective "bathroom" was revealed, that I had been hurled back through time to 1958, and I was standing in a chain-gang coop. I think I even checked to see if there was a chain on the bed. As I continued scoping the room, I also noticed the absence of a shower.

"Where is the shower?"

"There are no showers in these rooms."

"How do I, you know, clean up?"

Tracey said something about sponge baths. I know she said something more, but my mind had already moved on. I remembered that during my college fraternity years, I once saw an adult film where candy stripers gave the guys special sponge baths ...with happy endings. A peace came over me about the lack of a shower. Candy stripers will take care of that. I could see myself with a candy...my reverie was broken by Carol's voice: "It's no big deal. You can give yourself a sponge bath."

I immediately realized that I had to make sure no one told Carol about the candy stripers, or she would drag me off the transplant list all by herself.

The most poignant moment of our tour came when Carol began to cry again. She was so apologetic. Tracey immediately walked over and embraced her. Carol was already hurting, and I did not see things getting better from there.

# Chapter 5
# 2.1 And Counting

After some juggling of dates, I was scheduled to enter Johns Hopkins in mid-August 2012, to wait for a heart transplant.

On the day we were to show up at the hospital, Carol and I lay in bed, quietly holding each other. It was not based on a sense of finality. Far from it. Still, neither of us was ready to let go. Even with the lingering, we got up much earlier than we needed to for our late-morning admittance time. Carol busied herself packing a small suitcase with clothes I might want to wear for the first part of my stay—pjs, shorts, underwear, T-shirts, sneakers, and so on. I was busy gathering office items. I planned to reconstruct my office in my room so I could keep working. It is amazing how naïve we can be about things we have never experienced. When I was finished, I went downstairs and sat in my big recliner. There are times when you really should not do the routine. I got very melancholy. My basic thought was reasonable: Would I ever sit in this chair again? Would I ever sit here again while Carol and I watch *As Time Goes By* and smile at our similarities to the story lines? It was hard to grasp that we were going to leave our home and that Carol would be going back there alone…to wait.

We were pretty quiet on the ride to the hospital.

We arrived shortly before the appointed time. As you can imagine, we went through a pile of paperwork. Finally, we were escorted to my room. In no short time, there was a frenzy of activity surrounding me. When the medical team was finished, there were wires and cables everywhere. I looked like a full-blown scientific experiment, prepped and waiting for Igor to throw the switch. And that is pretty much the way I stayed for the next couple of weeks. I left my room only for examinations and tests.

During a tense time, there are unanticipated moments of generosity that bring a sense of relief. That is what happened when, during the initial couple of weeks of my hospitalization, our son, Todd, abandoned his bachelor lifestyle to stay with his mom. He helped around the house, even fixing dinner when he arrived home before her. He is a bit of a Spartan in his eating habits and diet. Whatever pounds Carol was losing due to stress, she lost even more due to eating like Gandhi. The fact is, however, Todd's presence was an unexpected blessing.

Once I was accustomed to my situation I, of course, homed in on the food. It was as good as the care. I had tacos, crab cakes, and other tasty favorites. One day I had a fruit salad that was not only delicious, it was beautifully presented. I wrote a note to that effect and put it on the tray. Later that day, I was surprised by a visit from the hospital chef. He brought with him the young woman who made the dish. He said she wanted to thank me for writing the note. He explained that that kind of recognition is rare. She was very gracious. I was humbled by the honor. It was during that stay that I was introduced to the TV Food Network and Ina, *The Barefoot Contessa*. When she would come on, I took notes so that when I was finally home, I could make some of her dishes. I became addicted to cooking shows. Fortunately, I was in the hands of a medical staff focused on something more important than Lemon Chicken.

The cardiac team attending to me was keeping me alive while we all waited for a heart. Of course, there was still the kidney issue, hovering around like a stepchild, occasionally acting up to make sure it did not get less attention than the favorite child. Very complicated. But I was at Johns Hopkins and in the hands of excellent doctors. So all in all, things seemed to be under control. Then the always-dreaded X factor popped up. It was something called *creatinine*. The only time I ever heard a term that sounded like that, people were talking about blacktopping our driveway. Confused, I consulted WebMD.com for a definition. "*Creatinine* is a waste product from the normal breakdown of muscle tissue. As creatinine is produced, it is filtered through the kidneys and excreted in urine. Doctors measure the blood creatinine level as a test of kidney function." My creatinine level had to be at 1.5 for the transplant process to continue. Mine drifted between 1.8 and 2.1. There began a daily watch to see where my level was hovering. I think there were probably pools going on among the nurses and doctors on which day I would hit 1.5. I know my family had a pool because I was in it. The number would get close—even as low as 1.6. But it never reached that critical 1.5.

I had been in ICU for nearly a month when I was removed from most of my wiring and placed in a regular old hospital room. The monitoring, however, continued for that elusive 1.5 creatinine level. I was also monitored daily by Carol and, almost as often, by Ashleigh. They focused on aspects of my care that I merely accepted. My days revolved around food I saw on TV and food I ate. Their days revolved around working, worrying, and wondering what was happening in my hospital room and in my body. They need not have feared that I was alone. I was blessed with regular visitors. I delighted in their company. My friend and former colleague, Dick George, told me he came to cheer me up and wound up being the one entertained. A couple we are close to, David and Diana Schroedel, had all the reason in the world to pass on visiting me. I would have completely understood if they had never visited. One of their sons had been treated for cancer at Johns Hopkins. Sadly, he did not survive. How did they walk through those hospital doors again for a reason so unnecessary as to visit a friend?

In one of those lighter moments seldom found during a death watch, Dr. Russell was visiting my room. He mentioned something about the medication I had been taking at home. I gave him my usual blank stare and pointed to Carol. In an effort to keep me from screwing up my medications and killing myself, Carol, thank God, had taken responsibility for handing me my daily doses. All I did was swallow what I was handed and go back to whatever

I had been doing when she walked in. As Carol was answering the doctor's question, she volunteered information about the natural substances she had included with my daily medication. Carol and I had a running, let's call it a debate, about the veracity of "natural substance" claims. Well, it was as if I set up the doctor to be my straight man. He was not a big fan of the stuff. Especially in a situation as delicate as my cardiac condition. Ah, man, I lived for moments like this. I chimed in.

"See, I told you. All that natural stuff is poppycock. Those pills you gave me are probably the reason I'm in here dying. Isn't that right, doc?"

I got exactly the response from Carol I knew I would. She was furious.

"I can't believe you'd say something like that." Then to the shocked doctor: "I was very careful to read each label. And I always called if I had any question about the ingredients."

"I'm sure you were very cautious, Mrs. Clews," the doctor gently responded.

"Well, I was. I'm not some crazy—"

"I don't think we have anything to worry about. But, let's stick with the prescribed medications once Mr. Clews gets home. Okay?"

Carol, still not wholly convinced, agreed to back off on the roots and nuts. Not finished, I spoke.

"I swear, you're so easy to rile. You and your beloved natural meds."

Carol started to respond, then muttered something under her breath. The doctor, recognizing what I had done, graciously reassured Carol that her bent for natural supplements had done me no harm.

## MY HEART TRANSPLANT FOR YOUR AMUSEMENT

When the doctor left, I was still laughing. I explained to Carol that she needed to lighten up about this heart thing. Carol asked me if I wanted something to drink as she poured me a glass of rubbing alcohol.

One afternoon, about six weeks into my stay, Carol, Ashleigh and Carter were visiting when Dr. Russell came to my room. He was not the congenial doctor I was used to seeing. A decision had been made, apparently by a group in which he had little say, that I should leave Johns Hopkins. I got the sense that the double transplant I needed was not going to be performed. The doc used some expletive about the decision and, I think, maybe the decision makers. A pall fell over the room. However, the good doctor was not finished. He had called a fellow physician who held a position comparable to his at a very well-respected hospital across town—the University of Maryland Medical Center (UMMC). While he was explaining to us what he had done to make certain I was not hung out to dry, Ashleigh was on her cell phone, typing out a message. I watched. "I guess she's letting the rest of the family know the party's over." Actually, she was texting a cardiac nurse friend who worked closely with the very physician Dr. Russell had contacted: "Does your hospital do multiple transplants?"

"Is this for your dad?"

"Yes."

"We'll do as many as necessary. Ask the doctor to have his records sent here."

Ashleigh told the doc what her friend wrote.

"Don't worry. It has already been done. Mr. Clews is going to be in the best of hands."

## 2.1 AND COUNTING

And with that, I got dressed and left Johns Hopkins with my damaged organs intact.

To this day, my brother is still angry with the hospital for kicking me out without fixing me first. Of course, his anger is misdirected, although you cannot tell him that. I have heard several explanations for my dismissal. I am not going to list them here. If any of them are incorrect, I do not want to be sued. Whatever the reason, I got dressed, and we left like a group of refugees. And, like many of them throughout history, we were headed to an uncertain future.

# Chapter 6
# The Woman Who Did Not Lie

"Hello. My name is Erika Feller. We're not going to let you die. We're going to find you a heart."

I thought, "Man, she's really cute. If this were forty years ago and I were single, I'd have been all over her like a rash."

The doctor continued.

"And then, when you are better, maybe you and I can run off to some South Pacific paradise."

I was transported. I could hear the music. "Bali Hai, my special island…" My head was filled with the song, and I could see the two of us, young and in love, running along a white, sandy beach, her long hair flowing, my…

"Vince, the doctor's asking you a question."

It seems that during my reverie, the doctor had been asking questions that I was missing. The fact was, that my new cardiologist was (and is) an attractive, vibrant young woman. More to the point, she was a remarkably gifted physician who was the head of cardiac transplant at my new hospital. Dr. Russell had placed us in good hands.

Oh, one other thing. I had just met the person who would save my life. Carol could loosen the grip on her bone.

From that day forward, Carol and I met with Dr. Feller on a regular basis. We talked briefly about my time at Hopkins. I told her about Ina and the need to salt tomatoes. I believe she only feigned interest. Her questions tended more toward my general health history and specifics about how the cardiac issues were affecting my day-to-day lifestyle. And, of course, about my medication. "Dr. Feller, meet Carol." The doctor and her staff learned very quickly that after "How are you today, Mr. Clews?," the next question should be "Is Mrs. Clews with you today?" A "yes" answer to that question brought out streamers and confetti.

The visits to see the doctor were routine, at least on my end. Go in, sit, wait, and be ushered, at last, to an examination room. Wait. Wait some more. In other words, they were the usual doctor's appointments, no matter who the doctor. As I began to feel less well, I became less patient with the waits. I do not know what I thought I would be doing if I were not in that waiting room, but I was sure it would be something with more purpose than focusing on lost time.

One day, I became particularly agitated over the wait. I told Carol that I would be out walking the halls. "Someone can just come and get me when my turn finally comes." And that is what I did. I walked the halls, steaming. After a short time, I felt a hand on my shoulder. I turned, expecting to see Carol. Instead, it was Dr. Feller. She had found me and suggested we continue walking while we talk. And so we did. I do not recall what was said. But that sensitivity, that act of genuine concern, nailed it for me. Of course, there was also her promise to Carol and me the day we met her. From that moment in the hall forward, even if she kept me waiting for a whole day, Dr. Erika Feller was my cardiologist, period.

That same day Carol and I also met with a UMMC nephrologist, Dr. Charles Cangro, about my kidney situation. He concurred with the evaluation of his Hopkins counterpart that I would not need a kidney transplant if the new heart performed as was expected. Nonetheless, he set up several tests to verify the prognosis. There had to be absolute certainty that the doctors were in accord. Carol, still concerned that the kidneys could affect the final decision on my heart transplant, had one last question for the doctor before we left: "What if he needs a kidney transplant and no one we know is a match?"

Doctor Cangro told us that there were other options, like harvesting a kidney. I do not know what transpired between Carol and the doctor after that because I was picturing fields of kidneys hanging off short plants as stooped-over medical workers in white lab coats and surgical masks and straw hats moved along open rows, checking kidneys, pulling off the ready ones and throwing them into coolers. I kept that thought to myself. But later, I was laughing pretty hard as I shared it with Carol. She did not get it. I guess you had to have picked tomatoes for a summer.

By the time we returned for the next visit, the doctor knew everything about my renal system, from my weakened kidneys to what they did with my foreskin. To further acquaint himself with my fluid-retention problem, the doctor arranged a series of sessions very much like those I had gone through at Johns Hopkins—you remember, the ones where the pounds dropped off each time. Well, this one was a different setup. They did not shoot a diuretic into my veins. The pee prompter was introduced through a drip. And drip I did in return. I do not know why, but I lost only ounces at each visit. It was extremely frustrating. When they had finished the sessions at Hopkins, I was damn near svelte. When they started the treatments at Maryland, I was "ready-eddy" to be slim again. Never mind the medical advantage. I was going to be buttoning my suit jackets and have people telling me how slim I looked.

The treatment worked. But not enough. My jacket stayed unbuttoned. The fluid problem would not go away. My heart was too badly damaged to pump hard enough to be effective. I began to re-bloat and have the same old problems getting around. I found myself breathing heavily at the least amount of effort. I felt terrible. There were days when it all seemed like too much. In quiet moments, I wondered if it would be better if I just stopped the treatments and let myself die. At times like that I would now and again recall a time when my very ill eighty-one-year-old father was confronted with the choice of a complicated and painful surgery or dying. He told them to do the surgery: "I believe God wants us to always choose life."

It turned out, so did I. We continued to meet regularly with Dr. Feller. One of the things I learned was that she took as much time as she, or her patients, needed to make certain that the checkup was thorough and that all questions had been answered. I found I was no longer as put off by waiting my turn. I was still not happy about it but not as put off. We also continued our meetings with the Nephrologist. Regular testing monitored the effect my failing heart was having on my vulnerable kidneys. I felt like I was in one of those old black and white Laurel and Hardy movies, where they would secure one end of the piano on the steep steps only to have the other end slip. I was the piano.

Thanksgiving arrived as my health worsened. My extended family was at our home for the day. No one said it, but we all knew why. When we were all seated, we joined hands for the blessing. I asked my brother-in-law, Ernie, to say grace. His prayer began typically, thanking God for our many blessings. Then Ernie asked the Lord to watch over me, Carol, our children, and the rest of our family during the critical days ahead. He prayed that God would provide the heart that would extend my life. Then, of course, he said a prayer for the family who would lose a loved one and whose gift from that tragedy would give me new life.

I need to say right here that that prayer strikingly brought home a harsh reality: if I did not die from heart failure, it would be because the lives of one family, perhaps enjoying Thanksgiving at that very same moment, was going to be changed, suddenly and heartbreakingly, forever. Yet, in the midst of such grief, they would think of others. Amazing grace.

# Chapter 7
# The Man on the Platform

In spite of the bloating and the difficulty getting around, I continued to keep up with my work. Film director Robert Altman wrote about his post-transplant anxiety, "I was scared no one would hire me." That was how I felt about anyone finding out about my pre-transplant condition. I recall working on a project at the Pentagon. If you have seen aerial shots of the building, it is every bit as big as it looks—17.5 miles of halls. It felt to me that the weaker I became, the more of those miles I had to walk to get to my meetings. No one walking with me knew about my condition. My clients were either current military or veterans. All were in very good shape. We quick-stepped through those halls. Forget elevators. We used steps, the good old-fashioned way to get from floor to floor. I hardly ever spoke as we climbed the stairs, or as we sprightly moved from one part of the building to another. Everyone thought I was a good listener. I heard nothing. I was focused on getting a decent breath without them knowing I was winded.

Meeting the requirements of the work I was doing for the military became increasingly difficult. But there simply could be no giving in to the health problems. It was bad enough that I never served—4-F, physically unable to serve. Both of my knees had been surgically "repaired." The recruiter saw the scars on my knees and told me to get lost. It made no difference the reason for my exemption, I was in the company of Vietnam veterans and, in my mind, I would have been the draft dodger who never fought in the jungles of Nam. So I took deep, quiet breaths and kept up. I am damn lucky I did not have a heart attack right in the middle of the Center Courtyard. I could see the marker: "Weeny writer croaked here."

One or two of my most frequent, and closest, clients noticed my progressive weakness and asked about it. Dennis Reeder owned a video production company with offices on the second floor of a hardware store in beautiful Alexandria, Virginia. The ten steps to the office were outside the building. On hot summer days, they may as well have been the steps to the top of the Washington Monument. There was no raising my arms in victory at the top. I would fall in the door to the reception area and stagger to a chair. His staff would kindly wait for me to revive before we started any meeting. Kindness and concern among his staff filtered down from the devout Catholic owner. Another client, without spilling the beans to his clients, would discreetly make certain there was a place for me to sit as we arrived at each location. As far as I knew, he had no strong faith. Just a good heart.

My final freelance writer's meeting came during the winter of 2012. I was hired to write a script the client was hoping I also would produce and direct. He knew I was dealing with heart problems, but had the courage to hire me when apparently more and more of my other clients had disappeared. I guess some of them decided I would die before I completed their work. The organization this brave client worked for was headquartered about fifty miles away from our home. The drive to and from the initial meeting wore me down. I wrote the first draft and went back for another meeting. It was on the second floor of the building. My client, who had no idea how ill I had become, took the steps instead of the elevator. I could not believe it. Frankly, I was frightened. I followed him because I did not want to seem weak.

On the way up the steps, he was talking with a colleague, so I let myself fall behind. I could barely make it from step to step without grabbing the railing to, without betraying my weakness, pull myself up each step. It was nearly impossible. When we reached the top, I was completely exhausted. Suddenly, I could feel my bladder weaken. My body needed to release the fluid the extra pumping had generated. I asked to join the others after I made a "pit stop." The client said, "Sure. The men's room is just down the hall." I wanted to run, but because one side of the hall had open cubicles, I forced myself to maintain a normal stride. The closer I got, the less control I had. As I turned in the door to the men's room, it was gone. I began to pee. And I could not stop the release. By the time I reached the urinal, it was simply to finish. I stepped into a stall, bracing myself on the side panels. And I cried. I knew the fighting was over.

The only salvation to my current situation was that it was winter and I had worn a dark blue, heavy wool suit. There was no tell-tale sign of the accident. I used paper towels to blot my clothes, and myself, dry as much as possible. Then I pulled myself together and went to the meeting. I sat with wet pants clinging to my legs. The meeting lasted well over an hour. When we all stood up to leave, I let my overcoat hang in front of my pants so that no one would rub against them and feel the dampness. I drove home knowing I had no strength left for any more meetings. My work life as I had known it was over.

I once had a timid client who met Carol and me for a meeting in downtown Philadelphia. It was a cold, drizzling winter day. When that meeting was finished, we were to go to a second one in the suburbs. We took the rapid transit system, which required a long and crowded ride. At one point, we had to change to a second line at an above-ground platform, one without cover. It was still drizzling. The wait seemed inordinately long. The diminutive client became increasingly unhappy with the circumstances. Finally, she just let it go: "I'm cold, wet, tired, and hungry. I want to go home."

I had become the woman on the platform.

# Chapter 8
# ♪Party Pooper, Party Pooper♪

At this point, I was not only physically drained, I was mentally and emotionally sapped. If a guy had been doing motorcycle wheelies, even if at that point he was in my driveway, I would not have had the positive self-image to challenge him. The ordeal was getting shattering.

I continued to write, mostly for myself. And with the hope that I could sell something and bring in some money. Carol still worked. I do not know how she got anything done because she was constantly calling to make sure I was all right. The circumstances were much easier on me than on her. I knew I was fine—well, as fine as a dying man can be. She did not know how I was doing from day to day, from hour to hour. Actually, minute to minute. For all she knew, my body was slumped over my keyboard making a hundred rows of k's.

Carol's birthday is February 27th. I am not crazy enough to tell the year she was born. The 2013 one was, let's just say, a significant one. Real significant! When I was in Thailand in 1992, the queen was celebrating a significant birthday. It was the celebration of six decades. There were celebratory illuminations everywhere. It was a beautiful tribute. I loved the way they recognized the birthday of this beloved woman. She and her husband were revered. When we entered the country, we were each given a small card, which was also in each hotel room. It read, in essence, "We are not amused by disrespectful comments about our Queen." Something about it also said, "And we're not kidding."

As for Carol's celebration, it would have been nice to string lights everywhere, but we missed that birthday, if you know what I mean. Strings of lights or not, the kids and I wanted this party to be an especially nice one. We decided to make it a surprise. A bash. We contacted more than seventy people (I am not saying that was her age) from among her current and long-ago friends. We rented the big room at the best restaurant in our small town. It was a very good restaurant. And very expensive, I might add. At least by my standards. I could not wait for the party. It was going to be the bee's knees. We even were going to have those little roasted lamb legs with ribbons, the ones servers pass around on silver trays at piss-elegant parties. We sent out invitations and received mostly acceptances. We booked hotel rooms for the out-of-towners and scheduled a brunch for the morning after. Things were nailed down to a fare-thee-well.

On the morning before the big event, Carol kissed me goodbye and left for work. She still had not a clue about her party. I went to my desk to write. I had been working for only a short time when I noticed that I was consistently striking the wrong keys. I would type a sentence, look up (I hunt and peck), and see that what I had written made no sense.

## PARTY POOPER, PARTY POOPER

Some of you who have read to this point are saying, "And so?" Eventually, the screen seemed foggy. My hands were shaking. And I was not sure what I was supposed to be writing. I decided I should go lie down for a moment. As I walked to the bedroom, I felt unsteady. My legs were a little weak and felt tingly. I laid down to take a nap. I was resting when Carol happened to call for one of her "check-ins." Well, she did not just "happen" to call. From the first indication that I was having heart problems, she became haunted with the idea that I was lying on the kitchen floor, flopping around like a freshly caught fish. I was surprised she did not have cameras placed throughout the house to monitor my every move. I imagined her saying, "I see you. Why are you sitting on the toilet? Are you okay?"

Carol asked what I was doing, and stupidly, I told her I decided to lie down and take a nap. No amount of insistence would convince her that I was fine. What was I thinking?

"Stay right there. I'm coming home right now."

I protested, but she was not going to hear it. To be clear about the rationale for her concern, I almost never laid down to take a nap. I did that in my chair. And generally, I kept that a secret from her. Come on. The woman was at work, and I was taking a nap. I did not need to reinforce that I was a bum. I honestly believe that had I been thinking clearly, I would never have told her I was in bed. On her way home, she called Dr. Feller's office. Andrea, the nurse practitioner with whom we dealt regularly, answered. She told Carol to call an ambulance and get me to the nearest emergency room. Carol called me back.

"Stay in bed. I'm on my way home. I'm going to call an ambulance to meet us there."

Now, at this point, a sane man would have said, "Okay, and tell them to kick it up a notch. I think the sheet is turning into a body bag." Not me. I wanted no part of being embarrassed in front of my neighbors by having a screaming siren blaring and lights flashing in my driveway, even if my situation warranted it.

"I don't want an ambulance. No ambulance."

For some reason, in a moment of wild abandon, Carol complied with my request. Instead, she called Todd and asked him to meet her at our home. He did. By the time they arrived, I was so weak that I needed help to get down the steps and out to the car. Carol sped us to the nearest emergency room. I was there only a short time when they told her that I should be where my cardiologist was if there was any chance of saving my life. So they sent me packing. Within minutes, I was riding in a speeding ambulance, lights flashing and siren blaring, on my way to UMMC. Well, at least I was not embarrassed in front of my neighbors.

The next thing I recall was lying in an unfamiliar room. I had no idea where I was. I did know that it was not my bedroom and that the woman in front of me was not Carol. She never wore white after Labor Day.

"Mr. Clews, see the clock on the wall. Can you tell me what time it is?"

I looked at the clock and could not give her an answer. I could see that the big hand was around the four and small hand near the eleven, but I could not translate that into a specific time. Nor, when I was asked, did I know the date. I do not know what happened after that because I fell asleep. Or passed out.

I later awakened to extreme pain in my lower legs. I am talking about the kind of pain that causes you to yell. Loud. That causes you to scream for help. It felt like my legs were on fire, and people were putting it out by beating on my shins with shovels. Trying to find a position where my legs did not hurt was a Hobson's choice. If I let them move, even just a little, there was increased burning and intense pressure like they were wrapped in a giant, hot vise. If I tried to keep them in place, it caused painful Charlie-horse sensations. Whatever, if any, drugs I had been given were helpful but not enough to substantially alter what I was feeling. When I could think clearly, there was no "Dear Lord, thank you for this suffering to help me understand Job's faith and strength." There was a little bit more of "Screw Job. The guy was nuts. Get me more drugs." A minute of severe pain is an hour of agony. The sheet covering my legs felt like it was sticking to the burns. When my movement caused the sheets to reveal a leg, I was certain I could see my skin blistering. In summary, my legs were swollen, discolored, and in pain. At some point, a doctor—at least I think it was a doctor—came into the room. Apparently his graduate course on bedside manner was taught by the Grim Reaper.

"Mr. Clews, you are dying. Do you understand me?"

"Yes."

"Do you have an Advance Directive?"

I had no idea what he was talking about.

"Do you want us to take extreme measures to keep you alive?"

"No."

Had the fates been a second off, the rest of this page would have read "The End." Literally. But just as I thought I had sealed my destiny, Carol and Ashleigh walked in.

"What's going on here?"

"Mr. Clews was just telling us that he wants no extraordinary measures taken if he…"

"Oh, yes, he does."

It was like being in the doctors' offices all over again. Never mind me. I am just the guy in the corner who only wanted to get home in time to watch reruns of *The Rockford Files*. Right then and there the two adults took over the discussion. Apparently I was wrong. I *did* want the doctors to take extreme measures after all. I could see that I had no say in any of this. So I just passed out.

Back at the ranch, Carol's party for the next day was, of course, cancelled. Let me say here that my family—my daughter in particular—still holds me responsible for ruining Carol's special day. Apparently, the reason for my collapse was what they consider "your irresponsibility." Looking back, I can see how they might see it that way. Let me explain.

## PARTY POOPER, PARTY POOPER

Several weeks before the party, I had to have a tooth pulled. Going back further, twenty-five years or so before the dentist trip, I had had both knees replaced. Subsequently, I have to take antibiotics before and after any dental event that draws blood. Well, I had had a bloody time on the dentist visit. I got the *before-the-visit* pill dose right. Now for the problem part. I felt fine a day or so after the dental work, so I stopped taking the antibiotics. That was wrong. My gums became infected, and I got sepsis. We might as well get familiar with this term "sepsis" now. WebMD describes it as " ...a severe blood infection that can lead to organ failure and death." Seemed like overkill, if you will excuse the pun, for my botched dental follow-up. However, it turned out that my choice to not medicate *after my procedure* was a disastrous decision.

In waiting areas at the Baltimore airport where people from the party that never happened jockeyed for return flights, as well as at the hospital where Ashleigh and Carol sat anticipating word on my condition, I suspect there was not much "sympathetic concern."

# Chapter 9
# The Other Side of the Mat

Up until this point, the talk of possibly dying from my heart issues had been a step removed from imminent. Now the sepsis issue put me on the other side of that step. Suddenly everything had changed. I was standing on the Grim Reaper's "Welcome" mat. The medical team working on me was fighting to keep me alive. Those were among the times that I was fortunate enough not to know what was happening. For my family, it was not that easy.

"Mrs. Clews, you and Ashleigh may want to stay here tonight. Mr. Clews is struggling. He may not make it through the night."

I do not know, and hope I never learn, what it must have been like for those two special women during those long, long hours of waiting. They made calls to the family, bringing them up-to-date. Carol called our good friend, Dedi, and asked that the church prayer team be notified. Other family and friends sent out calls for prayer asking that people ask God to spare me but that, as always, His will be done.

Before the night was over, my system with, I am certain, the help of massive amounts of antibiotics, as well as other drugs, had ably stemmed the sepsis onslaught. At least, for the moment. However, the crisis was nowhere near over. Doctors and nurses took my failing body and coerced life back into it. That was good. After all, I had already ruined a nice birthday party for Carol. It was only fair that I live long enough to make up for that. Of course, there is this question "How do you throw a party special enough to apologize for screwing up the first one by being stupid enough to skip critical medications that result in a life-or-death crisis that drags people you love, particularly the 'birthday girl,' through hell?" I think the answer is a party I could never afford.

I lay in a bed in the Intensive Care Unit (ICU) completely incapacitated while the medical team aggressively worked to keep the infection under control. If anyone touched my legs, the pain was nearly unbearable. And they had to touch them a number of times each day. Both legs were now terribly swollen. Especially my lower legs, ankles, and feet. It seemed that my heart was doing fine getting fluid to my legs but not so great getting it back. How is that for a medical explanation? More formally, it is called "venous stasis." The *McGraw-Hill Concise Dictionary of Modern Medicine* describes it as "the pooling of blood in a particular region which, in the legs results in edema, hyperpigmentation, and possibly ulceration." Lucky me, I got all three. The edema made my lower legs look strong, like those in muscle magazines. Looking at those legs makes you want to be like that. Looking at mine, with the hyperpigmentation and ulceration, made you want to puke. A shocking difference. Because I was bedridden, I had no idea about their strength. But I knew I could not move them very much. They literally had become useless. If I had been a horse, I would be writing this from a glue factory. That my legs could not move almost did not matter. My focus was on the pain. Take away the pain, and for all I cared, my lower legs could have been as disproportionate as Popeye's forearms. For once in my life, appearances were actually less important than how I felt.

I spent the next two-plus weeks in the ICU with unrelenting staff attention which involved, I suspect, considerable fluid-letting and wound care. And, I suspect, a good deal of pain medication. I wish I knew what specifically was done for me during that time so I could better describe it and give the doctors and nurses who saved my life the kind of specific acknowledgments you will find throughout this book. Believe me, however, if I knew their names I'd wrap them in rosaries. Throughout the rest of this book there will be times when I write of suffering pain. I am certain that throughout the remainder of my hospital stay I experienced the kind of pain I felt during the initial stages of this episode. But it set the bar ... and set it high.

Eventually, thank God, I was relieved of a substantial portion of the pain.

One day I was told that I was doing well enough to be moved the Progressive Care Unit (PCU). A relatively common definition for this unit is "one that specializes in treating medical and surgical patients whose needs are not serious enough for the Intensive Care Unit but too complex for the regular hospital floor."

That's when my hospitalization radically changed. I think they call what happened a "mixed blessing."

"Good morning, Mr. Clews. Let's get you out of that bed."

Two sparkly young people had walked in and introduced themselves as my physical therapists (PTs).

I played dead. I wanted no part of anything else they had to say behind those little smiling faces.

"Mr. Clews, I've got some exercises you can do in bed. I want you to do them three times a day. And I'm going to check on you. Let's go over each one together. They're going to help strengthen your legs so we can get you back on your feet."

I guessed they had not gotten the message: "The man in the bed is dying. He is to be left alone to go in peace."

My mother used to say, "No rest for the weary." And here were people in my room to prove it.

I would try to do some of the exercises each day. As the slightest movement still hurt, I fell way short of their expectations. I quickly found out that PTs are people of little faith when it comes to trusting the word of their patients. Where I would stave off pain by minimizing the exercise movement, they would ignore the pain, as gently as they could, and push me to do more. Frankly, from my point of view, not very successfully. I guess I was wrong.

"You're doing great, Mr. Clews. It's time to see if we can move over to the edge of the bed."

Let me tell you how far away I was from moving my body to the edge of the bed. I still could not move my toe on command.

"You're in the wrong room. I'm just now learning to move my toe."

It turned out that my protest that I was immobile was wasted. They wanted me to get out of the bed and into a recliner-type chair they had pushed into my room. I guessed they had not gotten the message: "The man in the bed is dying. He is to be left alone to go in peace." It turned out that not only did they want me out of the bed, they had the impression that I somehow could slide myself over to the edge and make the leap to the chair. Had no one shared my medical records with them?

We finally settled on a starting point. I agreed to try to move my legs. And I tried. It hurt, but I really gave it my best shot. I could not move them. Not even one of them. If our minds atrophied as fast as our muscles, get a short-term fever, and in a week we would get lost in the bathroom. I could not believe that being bedridden for such a short time had me so weakened. Totally disregarding another avoidance effort, the PT people insisted that I was going to get out of bed. They began to move me. My drip lines were readjusted. The PTs, nurses, and techs pushed buttons, causing whirring noises. Suddenly, this huge swing-like mechanism was moving my way. It settled over me. In a matter of moments, very painful moments, they had me in the swing, and I was being whirred over to the chair. Then I was slowly lowered into it. I was painfully, very painfully, jostled around until the swing was removed. Suddenly, the "dying man" was in the chair.

"This hurts. I'm in a lot of pain. How long do I have to be here?"

"Let's just see how long you can stay there."

"Okay. I'm done."

The PTs, the nurse, and the tech smiled gratuitously and headed to the other side of the glass wall.

"Hey, wait. I'd rather die in bed."

"The chair'll do just fine."

I do have to admit, it was good to be out of bed. But it was not necessarily a pleasant "good," if you understand. I stayed in the chair until the PTs returned. It was probably twenty minutes. They "slinged" me back into bed. Each day after that, with the help of the sling and the staff I made the move to the chair and back to the bed. Each time we did it, I supplied more of the muscle, or motion, to get into the swing for the ride. As the week wore on, I was helped to the chair twice a day. Each time, the move was painful. But successful.

It was not long before the chair sessions began to be accompanied by the friendly suggestion that "we" try to stand up. Each time, "we" rejected the offer. Finally, the smiles were gone, and I knew the jig was up. During one of my chair visits the PTs put a walker in front of my chair.

"Okay, Mr. Clews, I think we've been sitting long enough."

That was followed by a boost to my feet. My hands were placed on the walker. My legs felt pressure and instantly pain. I held on as long as I could and dropped back into my chair. The pattern continued each day, twice a day. Soon, with support, I could hold onto the walker and sustain myself for a moment or so.

"Why don't we try to take a step today?"

Because I was nothing if not compliant, I tried to lift my foot, but it was stuck, and that was it.

"That's okay, Mr. Clews. Don't worry about lifting it. Just slide it."

I could not move it. Not at all. My leg muscles did not have the strength to move my foot an iota. I felt like I was going to move it. It was as if my muscles were flexing to make that little thing happen that were required for the move. But no deal. The more I tried, unsuccessfully, the angrier I got.

"There's no way the damn thing's going to move. This is completely demoralizing. Just get me back into bed and leave me alone. Why don't you just go on and get out!"

I like to think I have handled adversity better. The PTs were gracious and overlooked my outburst. They had a job to do. They were gently persistent. The pattern, beginning by making me stand, became a part of my daily, albeit unwanted, routine. However, the lack of strength and the pain just made it impossible to do as they requested. Over the ensuing week or so, the pain began to subside. As it did, I became less resistant to the PTs' effort to get me out of bed. The swing became unnecessary. With help, I could slide to the edge of the bed. Then I could get into the chair, again, with help. I could stand with the aid of my walker, but I still could not walk. I was given more exercises to do in bed to help rebuild my deteriorating muscles. And I did them.

"Good morning, Mr. Clews. How are those exercises going? Shall we see what you can do? I'm betting on a big day. Where's that walker?"

"It walked for an ice cream."

The PTs were patient, but persistent. With the walker in front of me, I was again on my feet, attempting to move just one foot. And it moved. Just a tad, but it moved. It was really a slide. But look at me. My foot slid! The PTs tried, in their gentle way, to get me to push myself and move the foot farther. It just would not move. Not a fraction more. They recognized that, in my now immobile world, I had had a huge success. I wish it had been as exciting for me as it was for them. What I saw in my self-pity was a guy who had been a runner, now relegated to finding accomplishment in sliding one foot one inch. Any failed attempt to slide either foot further almost always ended with me back in my chair, sometimes even my bed. Relief and sadness. What a combination.

On what turned out to be my last day in Intensive Care, I was helped out of my chair, a walker was placed in front of me, and one last time, of course, it was suggested that "we" try that second step. Surrounded by the PTs and the tech, "we" tried. It worked. I took the step. I felt like Neil Armstrong. "One giant leap for mankind." I have to say this: if you have never been unable to use a limb, you cannot imagine the joy in even a little victory. However, apparently for some people, that is not enough.

"Let's try one more step."

"Why don't you try it, and I'll wait here."

They encouragingly pushed me to give it a try. I did. I tried. But the lack of strength and the pain just made it impossible.

Back in the Golden Age of the old black and white television, there was a series called *The Life of Riley*. Chester A. Riley was a blue-collar worker with a family. On every show he wound up in some confounding situation, usually of his own making. However he got there, once there he would look at the camera and say, "What a revoltin' development this is."

What a revoltin' development this was.

# Chapter 10
# It Ain't Dancing, But It'll Do

My need for more intense rehabilitative work led the hospital to move me to the Kernan Rehabilitation and Orthopedic Hospital. You have seen, and will continue to see as this story unfolds, that there were pleasant surprises along the way. Kernan was one of them.

For the first time since my hospitalization, I shared a room. Double occupancy. Our beds faced each other foot to foot, with drawback curtains surrounding each bed. There was one shared bathroom. One room, two beds, two curtains, and one toilet. Oh, yes, and two wheelchairs. One chair by each bed, but each one protruded into the other fellow's area. I think the space was designed to make patients uncomfortable so we would work hard to get the hell out of rehab as fast as we could.

The good news: I was treated like I had just checked into a nice hotel. They made sure they answered any questions I had. What am I saying? Any questions *we* had. It was still me, sitting quietly listening, or maybe not, in my corner of the room. I waited for my part.

"What's the food like here?"

It was as if the admissions people had been following us around for the past several years. They knew the drill: look at Carol, shake their heads along with her, and continue their conversation without me. I was becoming the invisible man whom no one needed to hear speak. I had visions of returning to church, and we would reach the part of the service where the congregation prays aloud in unison. And the priest would say, "Not you, Vince."

It was mid-afternoon when we arrived. There was the usual checking-in nonsense. By the time I was actually a full-blown member of the Kernan body, I had missed lunch. They gave me a pack or so of crackers with peanut butter and a carton of milk. I checked the TV to see if it carried MeTV, The Western Channel, and Lifetime (*Frasier*). I always dealt with the important matters first. They were all there. Carol was thrilled for me. She read Kernan literature while I watched TV. After some time had passed and she knew I was comfortably ensconced, Carol said she was leaving, kissed me goodbye, and actually left. Amazing. How can someone leave right before Perry Mason makes the murderer confess? But that is Carol. I will say it again: I love her. I could not wait to be back home with her. It was already turning into spring. The leaf buds were starting to appear. I was ready for robins. Then, just as I actually saw a robin, it snowed. The trees had snow on their branches. Not a lot. Just enough to be discouraging.

I was staring out of the window and continuing my rehab pity party when they brought in dinner. It was a hot dog and beans. My spirits rose. "Are you kidding me? I love hotdogs. Am I in heaven instead of rehab?" I decided that they did not know about my special low-sodium diet. And there was no way I was bringing it up. There were several sheets of paper on the tray. They were menus for the next few days. They read like a restaurant menu. Choices. All kinds of them. Things I liked to eat. Suddenly, I forgot that my legs were still swollen. Even the pain seemed ameliorated, to a degree. Gone was the memory that I was there because I could barely take a step and, without help, would get even weaker. I had real food to eat, and I was going to focus on that. Life was good. After dinner, I watched TV. Around ten o'clock, I turned off the lights. It had been a long, exhausting day, and I fell asleep very quickly.

Suddenly the door opened, and the opposite wall fluorescent lights came on. A man was wheeled into "my" room. He was accompanied by a nurse, a tech, and one or two other people. He was pushed to the bed on the other side of the curtain. He was loudly protesting being there. I mean, loudly. The nurse apologized and pulled my curtains shut. "Oh, good, the curtains are shut. That'll take care of the noise. I'll just go back to sleep." The yelling got louder as my new roommate raised his voice even more. He yelled at the nurse, the tech, and the people with him. A woman was yelling back.

"George, let's get your hearing aids in. George, listen to me. Where are your hearing aids? George, look at me. Your hearing aids, where are they?"

So that was the reason for the noise. I got it. By the grace of God, the devices were finally found, and the volume dropped considerably. But I was awake. "Hello, *Thriller Theater*."

The next morning after a good breakfast, I brushed my teeth, washed (in bed), and waited for the next move. While I was waiting, I was surprised by a visit from a fellow church member. It turned out Bill was on the Board of Directors of the rehabilitation center. He had been attending a meeting and stopped by to see me before he left. He brought the Director of Kernan with him. Nice fellow. A great gesture by my friend. From that day on, I was special. When my wheelchair was pushed down the halls, everywhere I went palm leaves were thrown in front of it.

Any illusion I had of importance was quickly dismissed when a therapist came into our room and told me that it was time to go for a session. I thought, "They'd better be talking a healing one." He was not. Not in the church sense of the word. I was going to my first rehabilitation treatment. I was helped into the wheelchair. He pushed me to the door and said, "Okay, Mr. Clews, let's go on down the hall this way." I waited. He matter-of-factly continued, "You go ahead, and I'll walk with you. It's the second door on the left."

The communication gap between the hospital and the rehab staff was getting serious.

"I just came here from the hospital. I'm pretty weak to do anything."

"I know, Mr. Clews. And we're going to fix that. Now, roll yourself on down the hall." With a gentle push, I was sent rolling. At the therapist's direction I wheeled myself into a huge room. It was filled with exercise equipment, exercise beds, exercise mats, and a few exercising people. I was lined up with others in wheelchairs. I waited for only a few minutes. A young woman approached me, pushing a walker.

"Mr. Clews, my name is Sandy, and we're going to get you on your feet."

"Well, I am certainly looking forward to the day I can do that again. But it is going to be months before I can…"

"Okay, I'm going to take this side, and Bob is going to help lift you."

"Oh, I guess you haven't heard. I can't stand …"

Before I could finish my sentence, I was out of the chair and holding onto a walker for dear life. And on my feet.

I don't know what those folks did, but the next thing I knew, I was pushing a walker, sliding one foot in front of the other. Sliding baby slides. But I was moving. Yesterday I could barely move one foot, and today I was "walking," albeit with a great deal of help. At that moment I felt like one of those people some TV evangelist hits on the head who then falls down, gets up, and is free of constipation. It was an exhilarating moment.

I returned to my room tired but feeling accomplished for the first time since I entered the hospital. I had walked. After a hearty lunch, the therapist returned to guide me to my afternoon session. As the week progressed I was able to do very uncertain sliding, always with a walker. The goal was to get around half the room on a track that circled a set of cabinets. I would venture out a little bit at a time, always with a PT or tech at my side. They were taking no chances.

One day, Carol brought me a reward for my work. Because walkers were in short supply at the rehab, sometimes affecting the length of my sessions, Carol bought me my own walker. She had even taped a piece of paper to the crossbar with my name on it. My walker, with an identity note on it, was the only one like it. I was reminded of the time in my high school years when we lived in the wonderful town of Hancock, Maryland. I spent a summer working in tomato fields on long, hot, humid days. The first part of the summer, I hoed weeds. Then, as the tomatoes ripened, I was down in the dirt picking them. It was ugly. Picking those tomatoes off the vines took a lot of back bending. It would take a while for my back to feel normal again. I worked with men from south of the border. I know because I was the only person whose first language was not Spanish. On the evening of my first day, my mother asked what I did for water.

"Oh, that. Well, there's a big metal barrel of water on the truck, and we all drink from it."

"From the barrel?"

"There's a tin cup hanging on it, and we all drink from it."

Now, I have to say here that my mother was not a snob in any sense. When she came from Italy at age eight, she did not speak a word of English. She worked hard, assimilated, and graduated from a big Washington, DC, high school Valedictorian (he proudly inserted) of her class. And that was the extent of her formal education. When she met my father, she was selling socks in a 5-and-10-cent store. Not a snobbish, blue-blood occupation. But now, she was horrified beyond belief that I was sharing a cup with a bunch of strangers. We didn't even drink from the same glasses at home. That night, she walked up to the local Ben Franklin 5-and-10-cent store and bought one of those little plastic thing-a-ma-jigs that, as it was pulled up, grew into a cup, then folded back down again so it fit in my pants pocket. She told me to use it instead of the company cup. I did. One evening, as we sat at the dinner table discussing my day, my mother asked for my cup so she could wash it. I pulled it out of my pocket to hand to her. My father, who had worked hard, blue-collar jobs to get through college and seminary, grabbed the cup.

"What's this?"

"Mom gave me my own cup so I don't have to drink from the same cup the other guys do," I replied innocently.

He opened the cup, wrapped his hand around it and crushed it.

"Confound it, woman, this boy will drink from the cup the other workers do."

That story flashed before my eyes as I looked at my very own walker.

Every day at rehab I went to the big room and was guided through a series of exercises. Over and over. Every exercise, every day, twice a day. The same old ones and then new exercises, harder ones. Often painful. Working through pain. I had never had any experience like it. Hard work and practice, I got stronger and, as it became less painful to move my legs, I was more comfortable moving further around a walking loop in the room. Always with the walker.

Always sliding my feet. It was time for the next step …well, first.

It happened one day when I was helped from the walker onto a wooden walkway with bars on each side. Once I was securely on the walkway I held on to the bars to steady myself. I did not move. Frankly, I was scared. My legs felt weak. But here I was, upright without my walker. I was told to hold the bars and slide my foot. I cautiously moved it until it was in front of me.

"That was fine, Mr. Clews. Slide it back. Now, brace yourself on the bars and this time try and lift, just a little."

I tried. I could feel everything flex. But, nothing. "What am I afraid of? I know I can do this. Lift. Lift." I concentrated. My left foot lifted. Just a little. It was off the wood. "Move it. Move it now." I moved it forward in the air. Just a little. I took a step!

"Excellent. Hold the bars and lift the right one now."

I lifted and moved the other foot forward. And then I took another step. I walked.

As I moved down the bars I used them only for gently steadying myself. I kept wanting to yell, "Look at me! See what I'm doing here." I was especially excited about showing off to family and friends—or anyone, for that matter, whoever was there to watch. Victory. Victory. I had almost forgotten how such a simple thing could cause such joy.

At times, my roommate and I, who were on different session schedules, would pass in the hall … still on our walkers but improving. We would give each other a smile and share an encouraging word. Every day we were getting stronger. And more neighborly. He and his family turned out to be very gracious people with whom Carol and I often shared company. After a short time, he left and his bed remained unoccupied for the remainder of my stay. Made me wonder about my reputation as a roomie.

Carol visited me every day. That was no small feat. The rehab was a 180° drive around the city from where she worked. Once again, she was driving a very busy beltway for that hour-plus drive to work, worked, then drove the same distance-plus to the rehab, spent an hour or so with me, drove an additional half hour to forty minutes home, worked on routine house and personal items, had dinner, went to bed, and continued the same routine for the time I was at Kernan. My challenges seemed elementary compared to the rigorous schedule she was keeping. I took a step, then rested. She was on a daily eighteen-hour merry-go-round…with no jolly music.

My therapy sessions were working, and I was getting stronger. Soon my walker and I were perambulating the perimeter of the exercise room with ease and, I might add, at a good clip. I was beginning to refer to Kernan as "Miracle Manor." I could not wait to wheel (I still had to use my wheelchair in the hall) myself down to the "big room," set up my walker, take my walks, and then do the exercises that were increasing my strength. Strutting my stuff. Well, strutting may be a little bit of an overstatement. But, compared to where I was when I arrived, there were peacock feathers broadcasting from my ass.

There were many somber moments amid all the joy. They were not about me. They were about some of the others who shared that rehabilitation room. So many were in terribly bad shape. Missing limbs. Paralysis to one extent or another. Broken bodies that no amount of exercise was going to make whole. All there for therapy. All giving it their best. Sometimes I felt that by merely using the same space, I was trivializing the very concept of "rehabilitation." I am ashamed to write that my sensitivity to others was too many times overcome by the joy of my own progress.

When I was not working with the physical therapists, I spent time in Occupational Therapy (OT). When I first heard the latter term, I assumed that they thought I needed to be retaught to be a writer. I was fairly certain that I had not lost my writing skills. The therapist graciously explained to me that I was an idiot. OT was not only about work. It also was about relearning how to handle everyday activities, such as brushing my teeth, getting in and out of the bathtub or shower, and getting up off the toilet. I could still do all the things they mentioned by using their assistance or hand bars for support. I was one of the fortunate ones.

One day the OT asked me what I liked to do at home in my spare time. "Sit on my ass, watch TV, and wait for the old lady to get home from work and fetch my dinner." That is another one of those answers I thought would be funny but dared not say. Instead, I said that I sometimes liked to cook. She took me to a kitchen just off the exercise room and asked me if I would like to cook one day and what simple dish I might like to prepare. I said, *pasta puttanesca*. Very few ingredients. Easy to make. I learned it from watching the cooking show *Extra Virgin*. Near the end of my rehab stay the OT found a fellow inmate who liked making homemade pasta. So she put us together to make *pasta puttanesca* with fresh pasta. A very forward-thinking therapist. It was a great moment in my rehabilitation. The entire exercise room smelled like my Italian Uncle Jimmy's basement...from which he bootlegged homemade wine and black market Italian package goods.

By the time my stay at Kernan was up, I was absolutely convinced that, if they would have let me, I could have walked to the car, with my walker, of course, and driven home. They had not been able to fix "delusional." I was leaving Kernan because they had done all they could do for me. My legs were still swollen and still inclined to building and holding a dangerous amount of fluid.

I was going back to the hospital.

# Chapter 11
# An Aging Pachyderm in an Open Gown

The return to the hospital was disheartening. I was so certain that I would have been home that being back in the hospital was emotionally devastating. I just wanted to go home, just live a normal life. It seems I forgot that I was in the hospital because I was extremely ill. As much love as I would have gotten at home, love was not the elixir I needed right then.

When I returned to the hospital, I was sure I would find yellow ribbons and banners reading "Welcome home, sojourner." It turned out that the staff decided against banners in favor of investing their energy on renewed efforts to release the fluids my body was holding. My lower legs were still swollen and painful, especially to touch, though not nearly as much as they had been early in my first stay at the hospital. I was put on a heavier dose of diuretics. The plan worked. I peed more but not enough. Part of the holdup was my fault. I learned about my patient rights. I was particularly drawn to the part that said that a patient had the right to reject treatment. So, after several nights of having my sleep repeatedly interrupted to go to the bathroom to pee, I refused to take the dinnertime diuretics. It worked. I could sleep through the night. However, it also meant I was retaining additional fluid. One day Dr. Feller took a few minutes to talk with me about my refusal to take the evening pills. She agreed that it was my right to decline them. She was an advocate for patients' rights. However, she explained, nurses are not kindly disposed to difficult patients. On the other hand, compliant patients make their jobs easier.

"It is good to be known as compliant."

I got it. I had let that idea slip away. But I was going to bring it back. And I did. Today, if you look at my records, I suspect "COMPLIANT" will be written on every page. But, sadly, not the word "slim." Once again, fluid was making me look like a Butterball turkey.

I once again had a room all to myself. And that, of course, makes you feel special. And I was right to feel that way. I was special. And so was every other patient on the ward. We each had a single room. Each of us was critically ill, and each was vulnerable to infection. In short order, I was gowned and in bed. There are some things that just seem wrong, no matter how much experience you have with them. Hospital gowns are in that category. There is nothing natural about being in a piece of cloth that ties around your neck, is short and loose, has no back, and that you are expected to wear with nothing under it. Even if it has flower or bunny designs on it.

"Excuse me. I think I'd like to wear some underwear here."

"I'm sorry. You can't wear anything under your gown."

"This is a little awkward. Very loose. Hell, in this thing I might as well just be naked."

"Yes, that's the point. Don't worry. I won't see anything I haven't seen before."

It seems to me that a female nurse developing such a blasé attitude about seeing a man's package must do wonders for connubial excitement. My father, who was a very modest man and hospitalized a number of times, once told me, "One thing I just can't get used to about being in the hospital is that you have to leave your dignity at the door." Boy, did he get that right.

My increasing girth reminded me of my only starring role in College Theater. I once had the lead in a Theatre of the Absurd play called *Rhinoceros* by Eugene Ionesco. I think that was my only lead in four years of theater. During the play a man turns into a rhinoceros. I guess that is why they call it "absurd." I was not cast in the lead so much for my performance skills. I was the fat guy in the theater group. Frankly, I had no idea what the play was about. If the people attending the show were depending on my performance for understanding it, they left completely baffled. But I perfectly filled the role as the fat, green guy with the horn. The director who cast me then, and hated my performance, would have loved my rhinoceros now. No matter how much diuretic therapy they gave me and how little fluid I was allowed to drink, my increasing size did not abate. Thank God those hospital gowns are made to fit an aging pachyderm.

Carol continued her daily visits. Ashleigh came almost as often, usually with some little low-calorie snack. Friends came by to cheer me up and provided encouraging words like, "I would not worry about your size. You've always been able to carry your weight well." Or, when I worried about what I was going to wear that would fit, "Goodwill has a whole gut-and-love-handles section." Hand me the green makeup.

Actually, there was another reason beside the diuretics that I should have been losing weight. During the night, I would wake up with an upset stomach. It was painful and kept me from sleeping. When I was a kid, say junior high school age, my brother and I had a couple friends we hung out with a lot. Sometimes we would eat dinner at their house. The parents were nice people, and we liked being there. The father was a strapping guy, very muscular. He worked in the local brickyards. I remember him as always wearing what was commonly called a "wife-beater" T-shirt, a term that had no relationship to their very happy marriage. I recall one night when he came outside after dinner and, from where we were playing, I saw him stick his finger down his throat and throw up his meal. He looked very comfortable with what he was doing and, when he was finished, wiped his mouth, smiled at us, and went back into the house. Yep, I remembered that.

So, one of those nights in the hospital when I felt horrible, I got up, went to the bathroom, and followed his procedure. I felt a lot better. After that, when the pain started, I prepared my forefinger for action and hit the bathroom where I would dispense of my dinner. No one knew. I did not have to eject the meals for very long. One day, Carol noticed that I was drinking regular milk with my meals. She noted that my chart should have read that I was lactose-intolerant. That item apparently had slipped through the cracks. The change was made to Lactaid milk. After that, I slept like a baby. The funny thing is that I knew I had a lactose problem and never thought to ask them to change the milk. It was another one of those instances when I absented myself from details that mattered regarding my health. Even now as I write this book, I still do not know what pills I take or when. Carol puts the right pills in the right slots in a pill container. She keeps me alive. I have often said, "If you find out that, God forbid, Carol has died, you can just order a second casket."

I was in the hospital for just shy of a month. During that time my legs lost some of the strength they had gained. And, some of the sores emboldened themselves again. I was beginning to get a familiar sinking feeling about my situation when one day they informed me that I was going home. It seemed like an eternity since I had annihilated Carol's surprise birthday party and turned her world upside down. That turned the screws tighter on her already complicated life by causing her to make nearly daily trips to the hospital, and then rehabilitation, while she worked a busy schedule in a job with abnormal stress. And, of course, she solely maintained our home. For her sake and my sanity, I was ready to be home where, perhaps ... perhaps, I could be of some help. The question was, however, was Carol ready to have me home? Considering the chaos I had created in her life, I was fearful that my soon-to-be homecoming was best described in the Robert Frost poem *The Death of the Hired Man,* where Frost writes, "Home is the place where, when you have to go there, they have to take you in…" Not very welcoming. I felt like I had been such a burden to Carol that she had every right to leave me in the hospital. It was not as if I was coming home healthy and we could move on with our lives. We knew I was going back into the hospital at some point for the heart transplant. And, until then, I was pretty much going to be an in-home patient. And she would be my caretaker. Not the Golden Years we planned.

# Chapter 12
# Carol, the Warden

The first thing I did when I got home was to head for my old, reliable recliner. I dropped into it like I had been shot. Carol sat in my lap, and we held each other. When she got up, I gave my attention to the other "member of the family," Sam's successor, Simon, our big old Bouvier. Now "member of the family" is in quotes because I am not one of those people who thinks an animal that lives with you has actually been granted "family" status. It is a pet. A subspecies. It chews with its mouth open. It poops in places that, if I did, would be a marriage-breaker. Simon, named after the now-late, great playwright Neil Simon, had been given to us when he was a pup. Carol loves babies, so that dog became hers from day one. But the dog and I had our own relationship.

I once owned a 1973 Volkswagen Thing. They were the tits. It was a bit beaten up, but I treasured the car. It was endowed to me by my very dear friend and employee, Billy Ezell, shortly before cancer took him, way too early, from a world of friends who loved him as much as did his family. The car was modeled after World War II German officers' cars. The convertible top did not go down; it came off and was stored in the trunk. The doors could be unhinged and stored with the top. The front window could lie down on the hood. In other words, it was like riding on a motorcycle without the fear of falling off. Simon loved joining me for a ride on any day when it was not raining or bitterly cold. We both liked the wind blowing around us and up our noses. I always admired his ability to do the latter without choking, which I always did.

Now, as I sat in my chair and stroked Simon's head I wondered when, if ever, we would be taking those rides again. I suspect he was thinking the same thing. I brought a special gift home from the hospital: open wounds on my lower legs and ankles. The skin on my legs was still taut and torn. Oh yeah, I was looking beautiful. When Simon saw the wounds, his floppy ears stood straight up, and he made himself scarce. Man's best friend.

My successful Kernan stay had strengthened my legs, but not so much that I could climb the twelve steps to get upstairs to the bedroom. I think I just heard you say, "Well, for Carol's sake, thank God. Who wants to sleep with a guy with open sores?" The answer to the question, by the way, is Carol. At her insistence, we tried several times. That option was gone. So, I stayed downstairs in my recliner. Sleeping in it was no problem. I was home.

In short time folks at UMMC had arranged for a hospital bed to be delivered, and it soon arrived. The family room was rearranged for the bed. It is not a very big room, so some furniture from there was parked in the living room. The once carefully-appointed room was transformed into a storage area. Carol was not real happy about that. I had always been allowed, to some extent, to keep the family room, shall we say, a little informal. But the living room? Neither the dog nor I was allowed to hang out in there. When the move was completed, the living room was unlivable. Only the couch and my chair were left in the family room, each somewhat hard to get to. To complicate matters even more, the only way to get to a seat was to squeeze, uncomfortably, between pieces of furniture or around the bed.

The rental "hospital" bed was not designed for patient comfort. The mattress was so thin I could feel the springs, way too well. The nights were rough, even painful. Ashleigh bought me a buffer that covered the mattress. After that, the bed felt more like a place to sleep and a little less like a torture rack. The head of the bed moved up and down, so I could comfortably sit up and read or watch TV. Ah, life was getting a little back to normal, if you discount being unable to navigate the stairs so I could sleep with the woman I love.

The skin on my lower legs continued to burn and, often, split like an overripe plum. At that time, the hospital had no program for continued home treatment of the kind I needed for my legs. So plans were made for another hospital to provide that service. The hospital was closer to home than UMMC. That was good. The chink in the plan? I could not drive. There was no edict forbidding me, just the understanding that it was not wise, considering I was not in complete control of my muscles to, say, move my foot from the accelerator to the brake. That did not keep me from thinking I might try. Carol had a different perspective on that deal: "There is no way you're getting behind that wheel. I'll call the police."

I thought that was a lot of angst over nothing. I could not even get into the car without help.

Carol took some time off to be with me at home and to get me to appointments. However, the need for her to be at the office would not allow her to be available as often as my frequent, and sporadic, appointment schedule required. This is one of the situations when family and friends are such a blessing. My good friend and lunch buddy, Griff, became a reliable source for transportation, even though he had to drive about forty-five minutes just to get to our home. And then another twenty minutes to half an hour to the hospital. We always stopped and got something good to bring home for a late breakfast or lunch. We loved to eat without, I might add, any regard for physical repercussions. Ralph and AJ were equally as ready to get me to my treatments. They were the ones I called most often when I forgot to arrange a ride and needed help on short notice. They were not eaters. But, oh, what delicious crab cakes they often brought for Carol and me, God bless their big hearts. Our friend, Patrick, also gave me rides to some of my appointments. He was studying for his deaconate, so he would bring weighty reading on faith to study while I was getting my treatments. I never knew if he was reading, praying or had simply fallen asleep during the long wait. Maybe it was some of each.

Michael, who kept a very busy social life, regularly would change his schedule to chauffeur me, even on short notice. We usually had late breakfast or lunch at one of his usual haunts. One of my favorite drivers was Ashleigh. We have a similar sense of humor. "Us and our crazy sense of humor." And tastes in food. There were still items on my "gastro bucket list." One was a real Italian sub. One day we bought a loaf of Italian bread. Because I wanted just the right bread, we must have gone to half a dozen places until we found the treasured loaf. We took it home and filled it with salami, provolone, olive oil, tomatoes, and onions. We would make ourselves one hell of an Italian sub. No bologna, if you will excuse the pun. Another item I had to have was Carol's best-in-the-world gazpacho. The veggies are not pureed. She leaves them in little chunks. We had that several times. One nice thing about being critically ill: people cater to you. It is not much of a tradeoff that I would recommend. Between family and friends providing rides, I never missed an appointment nor, I suspect, ever had to postpone one. I was the model compliant patient...except for the food.

There were two big nutrition issues I struggled with during this waiting period, and generally lost: a severe limitation on salt and a minimal fluid intake.

First, I was to cut my salt use to as close to zero as possible. "Doctor, we have a problem here. I am a Salter, capital 'S' Salter." I think the only food I did not eat without salt was tuna fish. And if there was tomato anywhere near the tuna, then I salted. For me, food without extra salt is food without taste. However, Dr. Feller seemed to be pretty adamant about limiting my use of the "enabler."

Carol and Ashleigh were big proponents of lemon as a salt substitute. So Ashleigh stocked me up with lemons.

"Lemons? What do they have to do with salting my food?"

Well, they had this cockeyed idea that squeezing lemon on food was a good substitute for shaking salt on it. It was as if they never tasted salt. I tried the lemon idea once. It ruined the whole meal. Lemon on mashed potatoes? If I had not seen the potatoes, I would have had no idea what I was trying to eat. But here is the peculiar thing: I did get hooked on eating the lemons. I ate every bit of the lemon, including the rind. I ate all of it. The way my friends would react when I took that first bite of rind, you would have thought I was eating maggots.

I did do something very mature for me: I sent for a low-salt recipe book. Some of the recipes even called for no salt. I responded to the information in the book by going to the website and buying salt-free or low-salt soups, crackers, candies, meat flavorings, beans, olives, pickles, salad dressings, and on and on. They had pasta, too. Pasta made without salt. There's a word for that. Oh yeah, garbage. I was also the recipient of a salt alternative that was orange-colored. I ruined one meal with that and threw it away.

In spite of all of my resistance to healthy eating, I really did try. I even made a loaf of no-salt bread. I gave the results mixed reviews but never did it again. Carol worked extremely hard to make certain that I was sticking to a low-salt diet and, at the same time, eating edible meals. That she pulled it off was apparent in my expanding waistline. It was not all fluid.

Restricting my fluid intake was much more complicated than I thought it would be. Most of my adult life, I had been like a camel. Six hours of tennis on a hot, hot day, and I drank no fluid. My opponents gulped water between games or sets. I did not even take anything with me to drink. Two humps. So I saw no problem with limiting the fluid until I realized how little I would be allowed to drink in a day: thirty-four ounces for the whole day. Carol found a plastic container just about the right size. She marked my limit and filled it with lemon water to the allowable point. It did not even fill the jug. That was it for twenty-four hours. You have no idea how thirsty you get during a twenty-four hour period until you cannot freely drink. It is a lot thirstier than thirty-four ounces will satisfy. Now, as you can imagine, I was thirsty all the time. No nice, big swallows of cold, refreshing water on a hot day. That minimized my water for later in the day. A second cup of coffee? At a price. A nice glass of wine with dinner? Not a thirst-quencher, so no. It was a trying and ungratifying time. Let me rephrase that. It was hard as hell to be on a restricted-fluid diet. That was especially true when I was at home where the turn of a faucet could bring sweet relief from thirst.

There was another problem with the salt-free and limited-fluid plan. It was a losing battle. I was sicker than it was effective. I continued to be engorged…and engorging more. I was back to putting on water weight. I did not like myself for looking like I did, even though I knew it was not my fault. Knowing that did not make my clothes fit. Nor my movements easy. Nor my clothes fit. And we know how I felt about that. All in all, I had experienced better times.

There was an incident during this time that was quite remarkable and did give me a boost. Carol decided it might be a good idea if I received a word of encouragement from a certain heart-transplant recipient. She set her plan in motion. It took several months for it to come to fruition, but it worked. She called me one day and said, "You're going to get a phone call. You won't recognize the area code, but answer it anyhow." So I did.

When the phone rang, I answered the call. The voice on the other end said, "Mr. Clews, this is Dick Cheney. Your wife tells me that you're going to have a heart transplant."

Carol had written to the former Vice President, who earlier that year had undergone a heart transplant. She asked if he would send me a letter of encouragement.

Instead, he called her and asked for my phone number. Our conversation lasted ten minutes or so. He wished me well, gave me his phone number, and asked me to call after I was home to let him know how I was doing. Now, if you think of Vice President Cheney as Darth Vader, that's fine. I do not. If you think of him as soulless, you are wrong—period.

The letter Carol sent to the Vice President is included in the Appendix to this book.

The worst part of any day was saying good night to Carol. We would kiss, and then I would watch her walk out of the room for the night. I listened to her walk up the steps to a dark room with an empty bed. She would turn the covers back for one. I wanted so badly to be there with her, to hold her as we fell asleep. Instead, we each slept alone, never certain what the morning might bring. But we were always hopeful.

"Mr. Clews. We're not going to let you die. We're going to find you a heart."

# Chapter 13
# The Best Piece
# of Advice Ever

In late spring, I was once again admitted to the hospital. Dr. Feller wanted me there because it gave the staff a better opportunity to deal with the persistent fluid buildup. I hated leaving home just when the daffodils were in bloom. However, they would be dead in several days, and I saw no point in staying put and joining them.

I returned for a second time to the third floor and the Cardiac Care Unit (CCU). This time, I got a room with a nice view of a small park across the street. It was a homecoming of sorts. While it was good for us to see familiar faces, no one really wanted me there.

It reminded me of coming home after I had been kicked out of the second faith-based private school my parents had scrimped to send me to. It was a small pacifist school in Virginia. At the end of the year, my father was told I was not welcome back—ever. So now I had been kicked out of two schools, no better for having attended either. As you can imagine, homecomings were a little less than enthusiastic. If the ward staff felt optimism about my returning in better condition, they shared a unique commonality with my parents.

The team immediately went to work. Once again, the goal was to get the extra fluid out of my system so that my heart would work better so that my kidneys would not fail. And so that I could live long enough for the transplant. The intravenous (IV) Lasix treatments were to begin again. I went into the hospital completely exhausted. One thing was for sure: carrying extra pounds made me feel like crap at the end of the day. As I have said, I was never a threat to men with that model look. That said, my normal weight was one I had gotten used to carrying. For some reason, I never adjusted to the added water weight. Maybe it was because pumpkin pie does not slosh.

The good news was that the treatments worked. I began to feel less like Falstaff and more like myself. Except for my legs. There were still sporadic open sores along my lower legs. I am not talking a little open spot here and there. They were big and getting larger. There were people in biblical times isolated from the rest of humanity for wounds far less gruesome than those appearing on my legs. Nurses were coming into the room in hazmat suits. Somehow, I overlooked all this when I would talk about going home, which I often did.

An aside as I write: From my open office window, I just heard a train whistle in the near distance. I had to stop writing and listen to it. I love that sound. Maybe it is my favorite sound of all those that inanimate objects make. I guess it is left over from my childhood when my mother would take me out each day to watch the James Whitcomb Riley train roll along the tracks through Francisville, Indiana. The train was named after one of the state's most notable writers, The Hoosier Poet. Among his more famous works was *Little Orphant Annie*, which later became the basis for the comic strip "Little Orphan Annie," which, of course, bred the musical of the same name. "The sun'll come out tomorrow." Funny how sounds can bring back such warming memories, especially ones with such an encouraging thought.

My painful, torn-up lower legs were beyond routine nursing care, so they were turned over to a wound-care specialist. Brent was his name. He became one of those people I could not wait to see. He had curative solutions he would rub on my legs, and the pain would be reduced. Not gone. Not even almost gone. But gone enough to make living with my legs acceptable. Here is something else he did: he worked with those big sores, and the little ones, with sensitive hands and a caring nature. He would tell me when something he was going to do would hurt and then apologize for hurting me. Sometimes I had to grit my teeth and hang onto the bed handles as he peeled the skin and dug pestilence and blight out of the wounds. Of course, like every other staff member and supplemental staffer who got near my legs, he wore rubber gloves. But let me tell you this about that: those wounds were so disgustingly gruesome that I would not have touched the person who touched the person who was in a room with a person who visited the person who was four times removed from any of them. Then again, maybe it is just me, but blood and pus make me queasy. Brent described my legs as looking like a cheese pizza with pepperoni after the slices of pepperoni were pulled off. Bad legs were his job, and he told us that mine were about as bad as any he had ever seen. Quite a compliment, that. He even took pictures of my legs to share with his medical colleagues. My guess is that you can find the pics on the internet if you are so disposed. Or sick enough.

When he finished each session, he would slide very tight compression hose over my lower legs. There were little toe holes so that the tops of several little piggies peered out. I guess that was for air. The hose helped keep fluid from gathering in my lower legs, which helped the sores heal. Fine. But it hurt when he put the hose on. It hurt while they were on. And it hurt when they were being pulled off. When they were not on Brent was working on my legs. And that hurt. I had to wear the hose 24/7. There were times when the pain from the pressure they put on my legs was almost as bad as that from the wounds. But here is what counted: what Brent did worked. The pain began to lessen. And the size of the sores began to decrease. It became exciting to watch them shrink and, one at a time, fade away. The large ones, maybe the size of a half dollar, would shrink to the size of a quarter, then a nickel, then a penny, then a dime, and then only a small hole was left. The length of time it took them to shrink varied with, as far as I could see, no rhyme or reason.

The largest wounds that were more the size of, let's say, Connecticut, took longer. Brent tried experimental treatments that sometimes helped. Imagine lying in a hospital bed, and the big event for the week is the arrival of the leg guy so that you could see how much smaller your open wounds had gotten. Bring out the party hats and horns. The largest wounds, one on each leg, took weeks into more weeks to heal. But Brent kept at it, even when he had to work around other nurses doing their tasks. Occasionally, I had a visitor or so when the time came for a treatment. I deemed that staying should be optional. Those who chose to stay probably still have trouble keeping food down when they think about the visit. I will bet they do not eat a lot of pepperoni pizza.

My lower legs still have large scars and bare, reddened skin from the event. They are so sensitive that even now when we are in bed, if Carol's foot touches them, I am awakened by the pain. Of course, I would rather have her there and deal with the wakeful moments.

One other note about this time with Brent. He was a man of faith, and sometimes we talked about that. It helped the sessions pass, with my mind on something far greater than where I was. I had the good fortune throughout the entire period of my transplant to get to know a number of medical staff who understood how God was using their hands to help heal my damaged body.

Now that I was once again in the hospital, Carol returned to the exhausting daily routine of home to work to hospital to home. Ashleigh also began making her regular crosstown battle with the traffic to return to the old hospital stomping grounds.

Every time one of them was there, I complained about the food. "The food sucks. They don't put salt on it, for God's sake. Bring me some salt. That'll at least make it edible."

Some years ago, I created and, subsequently, produced a series for Maryland public television, *Consumer Survival Kit*. After a year or so as a local series, it was picked up by the PBS national network. Each show was a weekly half hour of information on a single consumer topic. Home-buying, tires, cosmetics, funerals…you get it. Now, I am not the kind of guy who will do research before I buy anything. Too boring. So, *CSK* presented information for people like me. The material was couched in topical comedy sketches, song-and-dance numbers (I am not kidding), etc., all tied together by a host. It sounds nuts, but it worked. We even persuaded some notable celebrities to donate their talents. *CSK* was on air for about ten years. I left after five years, so I'm not exactly sure of the duration. The man I selected as host, Lary Lewman, became a mentor to me. His lessons were not just about television, an area in which he had many more years of experience, but also about life. At the end of production for each show, we would talk for hours. On one occasion, he gave me the best piece of advice I ever got, which I will now share with you for your edification:

"Get the world to treat you like its nine-year-old, and you never again have to do anything for yourself."

Carol says she will never forgive Lary for telling me that.

One of the blessings of this time was that, except for my legs, I was pain-free. That was true until the afternoon when my fingers suddenly began to cramp. It happened quickly and came out of nowhere. The cramping caused my fingers to go in different directions and bend to varying degrees, all at the same time. It was as if each finger was going on its own walkabout. The pain was excruciating. I had never experienced pain of that sort. And I knew pain. Worse, there was no relief. Not a thing anyone could do to help. The pain lasted for minutes at a time. I think you are supposed to pass out from pain like that. No such luck here. The event was—get this—the result of low sodium. Not enough salt. What was I trying to tell Carol and Ashleigh about salt? You remember. Remember when they insisted I use lemons instead of salt? There's no substitute for salt. Now my hands looked like bird claws with crippling arthritis. We need salt, a lot of salt. The pain continued for several days while potassium was introduced into my salt-starved body. God Himself could not convince me ever again to substitute lemons for salt. Lemons.

As the days passed, I got comfortable with being in the hospital again. "Comfortable" was, of course, relative. But there were nurses and techs responding around the clock to my every need. I accepted, always to a degree, that this was where I was meant to be, and I could adapt. So you can imagine my surprise when I was told that I would be leaving. "Already?" Frankly, I had mixed feelings about exiting the hospital with the fluid still there, with my heart still dying. And what about my kidneys? All the problems that caused me to be in the hospital were the same problems I was taking home. There seemed to be a flaw in that plan.

My fears were assuaged in a single sentence: "Dr. Feller ordered it." Medically speaking, those words meant the deal was on. I packed my bags. Well, Carol packed what little I had with me. I was busy waiting to see if Alistair was going to propose to Judy. Hey, we are talking a climactic moment on my favorite Britcom. Before I was able to find out how Judy answered, Carol had stripped me of my gown, thrown some clothes in my general direction, had my gear packed, and the nurse had a wheelchair at the door. In other words, I was not leaving. I was being thrown out.

In just over an hour, I was home in my chair. The dog was lying beside me. Carol was fixing lunch for us. It was utopia. Still, I was a little concerned about what had happened. This was what I knew of patients being sent home before they were well: they were sent home to die. There was a fleeting thought that maybe that was what was going on with me. Then I recalled the promise, "We're not going to let you die." That worked. Plus, the dog stopped asking for "one last ride." Once I settled my self-generated doubts and conflicts, I decided to create a walking program. The first floor of our house did not provide the track-like layout or distance my ward had. But I used the floor arrangement and space to walk each day, twice a day. Carol's presence invigorated me. I did not have to watch her leave every night except to go upstairs to our bedroom. Still my no-go zone. The ensuing weeks were dotted regularly with doctors' appointments. They were mostly cardiology appointments, but they were keeping their eyes on my kidneys, too. I provided regular on-demand blood tests and urine specimens. Blood on demand. No problem. Urine on demand. There was something disconcerting about hitting a little cup in your hand that turned it into a crisis. I knew God could not possibly condone that kind of stress.

My lower legs were still a mess. They were swollen with the remnants of the beating the wounds had left. Home became a hospital again. Two or three times a week, a nurse would come to the house and work on my legs, picking away parts of scabs or sometimes a complete one. She would treat what was left and the remainder of my legs with oil. When the insurance for that nurse ran out, Carol was stuck with the odious task of treating my legs. To her everlasting credit, she still loves me, even after that vile chore. A nurse came by on alternate days to give me my IV Lasix treatment. We would sit and talk while the line dripped, dripped fluid. And, just to ensure that I saw nothing of *Daniel Boone*, a physical therapist came to fill any other open time. Simon watched all these activities. He seemed never to get what was going on. I understood. I always felt the same way when he would lick what was left of his privates.

# Chapter 14
# No Rest for the Weary

During my home respite we met regularly with Dr. Feller. On more than one occasion, she reinforced the point that the success of the surgery and recovery would be affected by my strength. She "encouraged" me to exercise so my body would be as strong as possible for the onslaught. Now, this ongoing exercise thing was becoming a bit of a concern to me. I once read that Neil Armstrong, the first man to walk on the moon, observed this about exercise: "I believe that every human being has a finite number of heartbeats. I don't intend to waste any of mine running around doing exercises." Made perfect sense to me. My plan was to limit my exercising so that I would live longer. I do not think Dr. Feller was necessarily an advocate of the Armstrong exercise theory. Carol, also not an Armstrong subscriber, was hell-bent on making sure that we followed instructions we were given for our home stay. She got up every morning, got ready for work and came downstairs to where I was sleeping in my old chair. Sometimes we would have coffee together. That is when she would remind me how important exercising was for the surgery and recovery. Then she would fill up the quart jug with water to that damned line that marked my fluid limit for the day. She would point to the line.

"Don't forget, this is it until tomorrow. Drink wisely. And be sure to walk. If it were me, I'd do it at least ten times today."

"If it were you, I would not be telling you what to do."

I never knew who was more tolerant—me, for listening to all her instructions every day or her for, well, by now you know why. The fact is that every day, I did what Carol said. When you are holding onto life and the caregiver gives you instructions, you are pretty compliant. Especially when you love the caregiver.

While I was pretty happy being at home and trying to find reasons to stay out of the hospital, Dr. Feller, on the other hand, was working to get me back in. It was once again that old familiar 1-B, 1-A, 2-B, 2-A, and so on dance. I was aware that she was writing letters and going to meetings, urging that I be moved back into the hospital to wait for a heart. One reason I knew what she was doing is that I would get letters from the United Network for Organ Sharing (UNOS). "Dear Mr. Clews, we would like to inform you that your status on the UNOS heart transplant waiting list has changed. As of (the date), you are, once again, active on the heart transplant list as a status (status)." Then there was the reminder that the double transplant was still in play: "…and active on the kidney transplant list." I did not know why, but the prospect of the kidney surgery unsettled me more than that of the heart transplant. They screw up the heart surgery, I die. *Fini.* They screw up the kidney bit, and I spend the rest of my life peeing through my little finger. Or something like that.

One Sunday during this home stay, our parish priest asked me to come to the front of the church. Our church is orthodox Anglican, which I describe as Baptist-minded but love liturgy. Because we believe that healing can come through prayer, he asked the congregation to join him, surround me, lay hands on me, and pray for my healing. It was an incredibly moving moment in my journey. If you are thinking that the prayer did not work, based on the fact that I still needed the heart transplant, I can only write this: I believe God is quite comfortable healing through the hands of physicians and other medical professionals. That is fine with Him. He knew them before they were born. He often works through human intermediaries.

As long as I was going to be home for a while, I attacked my Gastro Bucket List again. I even made a second round on some items, like the Italian sub. Friends pitched in to help me fill the list. Ralph and AJ brought crab cakes again and added pies. Todd sprang for steamed crabs…without the seasoning. I was having fun now. Carol even made, albeit reluctantly, a couple of dishes that might have been on the "Do Not Touch" list. Sadly, she kept it to the "Can Touch, But Only A Little" list.

The ongoing treatments on my legs was helping eliminate some of the horror show they had become. My pain was not quite so severe. The home IV Lasix treatments were removing some of the fluid buildup. Of course, the treatments were a bit of a losing battle, but they had to be done.

The stress of the wait was getting to us. We were tired. Very tired. Especially Carol. How in the world does someone watch the love of her life physically failing and remain strong, much less stay sane? I do not know, and I never want to know. We decided that we both needed a break. Baltimore is only a few hours from Ocean City, Maryland. We liked it there. Here is how rest is medically defined: "Sit on a sandy beach on warm sunny days and watch the ocean waves lap onto the wet sand." That is it. Look it up in any medical dictionary. So that is what we decided to do—go to the beach. We also decided we had better let Dr. Feller know how to reach us while we were gone.

"Hi, Doc. Carol and I are going to OC for a long weekend. We'll have our cells with—"

"I'm sorry, Mr. Clews, you're not allowed to go that far away while you're waiting for your call."

"It is only three, three and a half hours away, at the most."

"I'm sorry. You have to be less than two hours away. If a heart comes in, we need you to be able to get here within an hour and a half."

The choice was hard. I voted for dying on the beach. We spent a long weekend at home.

In the middle of all of this mess, we celebrated Father's Day. My dad had passed away before all my heart trauma began. It was a mixed blessing. His strength and support would have been encouraging, a genuine blessing. On the other hand, he did not need to witness a son dying. He had had enough tragedy in his life. His sister died from pneumonia when she was four. Dad had a twin brother, George. When the twins were nine years old, they were walking along a road when a drunk (find PC in another book) driver hit George. He died at the hospital. It took years for young Gordon to recover. I recalled my last Father's Day with my dad. Now, I quietly wondered if this current one was my last for me and my children. My only clue that anyone at the table had any thoughts of that kind were the Father's Day cards. They were all from the "missing you" section.

Shortly after Father's Day, we received a call alerting us that efforts being made to get me into the hospital were bearing fruit. It seemed that an admission target date sometime prior to the July 4$^{th}$ weekend was looking realistic. I once heard that holidays are a good time to be on a transplant list. Celebratory times cause accidents, which create increased numbers of transplantable organs, ones that were not products of death by disease. There seems to be something wrong about thinking of holidays as an opportunity to "harvest organs." Unless you are waiting for one.

# Chapter 15
# Right Where I Needed to Be

On June 30, 2013, I was checked back into the University of Maryland Medical Center, where I would wait for my heart transplant. I was not nervous. In other words, I am not a fool. I am a complete and utter fool.

The admitting process, once again, involved an abundance of paperwork. The same questions seemed to be on each form. And, again, my signature was required on every page. I had this temptation to sign all of them John Jacob Jingleheimer Schmidt from the children's song of the same name. (If you know the song, it is stuck in your head now.) I was admitted to the Progressive Care Unit (PCU). I spent several days there while they made an intensive effort to reduce the amount of fluid I was holding. They were successful enough to make me feel more comfortable. More to the point, there was now a little more distance between hospital socks and a toe tag.

Because I now required less intense attention, I was moved to the Cardiac Care Unit. It was the old, familiar stomping grounds. There was a nurse's station and, maybe, ten rooms on a curve around the area. Once again, I had a room all to myself. There could be no room-mating. A cough from one man could turn the next man's bed into a casket.

Once again, (it is beginning to feel like an old story), the staff immediately went to work on the fluid issue. I was hooked up to lines feeding me diuretics. No drip. Right into the veins like an open fire hydrant. It did not hurt. Except for certain times when the stuff going into my arm caused a reaction. That happened on several occasions. The pain was terrible. It was very much like having liquid fire rushing through my arm. I felt like my muscles were being blown up to the point of explosion. That, in turn, caused a sensation that can be best described as having an extended total-arm Charlie horse. Even after the procedure was finished, it took a while for that pain to go away.

Carol spent a very active check-in day with me. She talked with the nurses about everything from the meds I would be taking to the food I would be eating. What an irony there is to our relationship. She was not sick but wanted to know what was going to happen. I was dying and trying to find out if the TV lineup included *Father Knows Best*. I was not concerned about what Carol was doing. She was there. The longer, the better. Thank God, she was in no hurry to leave. It would seem that Carol and I would have been seasoned and unfazed by our circumstances, having been through this opening-day routine before, several times. However, what we had learned is that nothing is certain. No one wants to be away from the one you love at a critical time.

Finally, check-in day drew to a close. Then she was gone. A pallor fell over the room. That never changed, no matter how often Carol left. You would think regular separation would make the sadness of parting less biting. It did not. Not in any sense of the word. An empty hospital room can be an incredibly lonely place.

The first full morning there, I was reminded that sunrise is mid-day to the medical staff. The nurse came in with a jovial salutation.

"Good morning, Mr. Clews. Did you sleep okay? Let me get your vitals, and then you can get into the bathroom to bathe up before breakfast gets here."

It was 5:30. How dirty did she think I got overnight? I did as I was told. As I was "washing up," I found that I could not stop thinking about eating. I finished, got settled, and waited for the food wagon. I was ready to eat well before its 6:30 scheduled arrival. It is interesting how hungry you become when you think you are supposed to eat at a certain time and the food comes later than it was scheduled to arrive. It arrived between 7:30 and 8:00. That first day was a pattern that seemed to be hospital policy. Whatever time the meal was supposed to arrive, it did not. It was always late. If they ran meal schedules in prisons the way they run them in hospitals, TV news would be showing a prison riot a day. When breakfast did come, the eggs, of course, were cold. I reminded myself then always to order cereal for breakfast. Cold cereal.

I have, unfortunately, been a somewhat regular attendee at hospitals. I do not recall having ever been well enough to give a damn about what the nurses were wearing. My main interest was that a nurse's outfit was not blood-spattered, especially with my blood. Blood on white is not a good fashion statement. However, this time, I did notice that gone are the days when nurses' outfits made them look like Herdies. Today's nurses wear multicolored tops with a variety of designs. Their patterns range from causes they support to images designed to take the attention away from the blood spatters on their uniforms. And they often are not baggy, at all. The nurses who attended me ranged from winsome to the stuff of which daydreams are made. One very devout person who visited me while some of the more "daydream" nurses were on duty later told Carol, "No God-loving man should ever be exposed to something like that." As for candy stripers' uniforms, I do not know if they look like candy canes because not one ever came into my room. I still suspect Carol's hand in their absence.

My room had a fairly comfortable recliner. Not as comfortable as the one at home. But fine for the moment. From that chair I could see the street below. I watched people busily going here and there, unrestricted by an inability to get around. They were walking to their eventual destinations without a thought to moving their legs. Sometimes the view depressed me. Not a deep depression. Just that wistful envy for what others could do that I could not. There were times that my lot bothered me more than at others. For example, watching the people I was watching who were sometimes going to sit in a ballpark, usually with friends, to eat a hotdog with the fixins', drink an overpriced beer, sing "Take Me Out to the Ballgame" during the seventh-inning stretch, "cheer, cheer for the home team," and then return past my window, vigorously sharing commentary on what the "manager should have done." If you are a ball fan, you understand why some days, my situation was just downright demoralizing.

At one point much later in my stay, I was visited by a member of the psychology staff. A very pleasant fellow, he asked me if I was depressed.

"If you are asking if I am perpetually depressed, the answer is no. If you are asking me if I ever get depressed, if I did not, you can just have me wheeled right behind you to your ward."

I had been there only a few days when Dr. Feller "suggested" that I begin walking every day, several times a day. She reminded me again that the success of the surgery and recovery would be affected by my strength. She wanted me to exercise so that my body would be as strong as possible for the onslaught. Now, this exercise thing remained a bit of a concern to me. I reminded her about Armstrong's comment about finite heartbeats. She still wanted me to exercise. I decided it was a losing battle. Cardiologist, exercise expert, and author George Sheehan wrote, "Exercise is done against one's wishes and maintained only because the alternative is worse." Because the alternative for me was dramatically worse, I decided to buy in and walk.

One day, I scouted the ward layout beyond my room. At one end there was a reception area with a door that led into a larger hall I knew only from a gurney point of view. The hall ran along a glass wall that overlooked part of the lobby, the part with the fresh cookie stand. I could smell them baking. At the end of the corridor, there was another entrance to the ward. Continuing from there to my door completed a hardy circular walk. All in all, it was probably a twenty-yard walk. That was going to be my course. I set a goal: build my walk up to ten times around, twice a day. It was a far cry from running six miles. But I was a far cry from the man who used to do that. I began the twice-a-day routine.

As I began to build the number of laps past four, I quickly found a flaw in the plan. I could not remember how many times I circled the route. Math had never been my strong suit. Nor, obviously, memory. The nurses and techs at the station tried to help me keep track of my loops. But the other confounded patients would call for them right during my walk. It was all very disruptive to the count. So I devised a plan. I tore ten slips of paper. As I began my daily walks, I carried them in my left hand. Each time I passed my room, I would move a slip to my right hand. My walks became a very important part of my day.

The daily plan for my stay was set. Each day started with a 5:30 wake-up call, ablutions, breakfast, walk, watch the "Beaver" and "Perry" while I did my bed exercises (which lasted about a week), make myself available to the doctors during rounds, eat lunch, read, watch the Britcoms, visit with guests, doctors and nurses, visit with Carol and/or Ashleigh, dinner, walk, read or watch TV, ablutions, lights out, get a good night's sleep, and start all over again the next day. Yes, that would work. Now, it was just a matter of waiting for my new heart and then home.

# Chapter 16
# A New York Kind of Girl

"Then home" was not the speedy "then home" I imagined it would be. I love the "mind over matter" gurus. "If you think you can do it, you can." Maybe it works... if you do not have to wait for a heart transplant first.

The biggest variable in my life was still my status on the "who's up, who's down" chart. At the moment, I was down. Riding between 1B, 2B, 1B, and so on. Always there was the big question: Had the doctor's attempt to make me a 1A succeeded? Carol was visiting one day when a nurse gave us the news: I was 1A. I was finally there! I was that next in line guy. Carol, overwhelmed with joy, broke down. Relief was letting itself out. The woman who would not let go of the bone was seeing the reward for her tenacity. I felt good for her, in a mixed-feeling sort of way.

Carol is a striking woman. She is attractive. She has a figure a lot of younger women would give their eyeteeth to sport. She is smart, active, conversational, spiritual, and hot-looking. I have never worried about her well-being if I died first. While she could take care of herself, I always felt confident that widowed, she would not have to be single long. Some guy with a lot of class, and as much wealth, more than I could ever provide, would snatch her up in a minute. Her life would be wonderful. She could move on. Her life would be so good that I'd just be "a memory on the far horizon." I told her all that once to cheer her up. Funny how people's perceptions can be so different. I saw it as a big compliment. I have had the good sense never to say it again. Okay, except here. And only this once. And with apologies to her.

I had not been back in the hospital for very long when my first crisis hit. I will try to be as specific as I can. I lost my green footies. Footies are best described as low-cut socks with flexible grip bottoms. I was given a pair as soon as I was admitted. I was instructed never to leave the bed without wearing them. Footies help restrict slips and falls. "Fall" is the hospital "F" word. It took several attempts before I was given a pair that were absolutely comfortable. They were green. In just a short time of wearing the green footies, they became perfect footwear. I wanted to make sure they were not lost in the routine change of sheets, towels, and so on. When they were not on my feet, I tied the green footies to the bed posts. My green footies became a critical aspect of the comfort of my hospital stay. I know this sounds crazy, but no other color fit as well. Everyone respected my quirk about my green footies. On one particular night, when I went to put on my green footies for a trip to the bathroom, they were gone. I asked the nurses and tech about my green footies. Nope, no one had moved them. I remembered that Ashleigh was my last visitor. And that was why I made a midnight call to her.

(Groggily, very groggily) "Hello?"

"Someone took my green footies."

"Dad, are you okay? What's wrong?"

"Someone took my goddamn green footies."

Propriety prevents my recounting her exact words here. Though she was right about where I left them.

While I was concerned about finding a secure place for my newly found green footies, Dr. Feller and her team were homing in, once again, on getting the new excess fluid out of my system. The additional fluid was not only taking a toll on my health, it was debilitating to my morale. I was locked in a body that was uncomfortable and, in a number of areas, painful. My legs, although much better, still reacted with pain to any significant touch.

The needles taped at intervals throughout my arms at several places were there to usher medicine in and fluid out. They hurt me any time I moved. The tape holding the needles in place tore at my skin if the needles or tubes moved. Or if I did. Getting those needles into and out of my arms was almost always painful, in spite of the earnest attempt by the nurses and phlebotomists to cause as little discomfort as possible. Sometimes, and more often than not, when the tape holding the tubes in place was removed, it tore away some of the skin. Always, of course, the hair on the spot wound up in the trash with the used tape. I don't need to describe the hair-pulling pain, do I? Perfectly placing the needle often involved moving it to adjust the position for the best flow of blood. Imagine a needle being moved around under your skin. And sometimes, the final placement of a needle was in a spot especially sensitive to any movement. An example might be a needle stuck in a vein that was stuck on top of my wrist. I would unthinkingly move my hand, and the needle attached to a tube attached to a bag attached to a stand would pull while the stand held steady. Sometimes, even the stand yelled, "Ouch!" My pain might be a boo-boo compared to the pain a guy down the hall was having. Nonetheless, his pain was not in my room. Mine was. In those moments, it was hard to feel empathy for anyone's pain but my own.

My blood had to be drawn numerous times every day for a variety of reasons I would not have understood even if they were explained to me. Every day. That includes a needle to start the day. Ain't that beautiful. My regular morning blood-letter was a particularly gentle chap, a black man whose warmth, personality, and good skills made the draw almost painless. Almost. I will say this: he was better at it than most of the other phlebotomists. In spite of the purpose of the visits, I looked forward to seeing him. We always chatted for a while each morning as he prepared for that morning's blood draw. It was about that same time Carol began to bring in some fruit and honest-to-God goodies. The goodies were my idea. The fruit, hers. There were always fewer goodies. At one point during this period I developed a particular yearning for oranges. And grapes. Not hospital grapes, but big, juicy, seedless grapes. One morning, my newly found friend brought in some of those grapes for me. He had purchased them at a fruit stand he passed on his way to work. I could not believe it. I should not have been surprised that this man would make such a kind gesture. He would often bring vegetables for Carol to take home. He never let us reimburse him. It did not matter how much we insisted, the answer to helping cover the cost was a pleasant but firm "No, thank you." I wish I had his name to add to this book, both in the Acknowledgments and here. I knew it then. Shortly after I left the hospital for the final time, we learned that he had passed away. What a loss. We cannot afford here on earth to lose such angels.

On a happy note, I am pleased to say that one day, much of—not all of—the pain of repeated needles was brought to a halt. Not a second too soon, either. I had gotten so many shots and blood draws every day that my arms had begun to look like the side of Bonnie and Clyde's car. They finally reached the point where no usable vein could be found. At that point, they put a peripherally inserted central catheter (PICC) into my arm. From then on, the needles were inserted into the PICC instead of directly into my arm. Unfortunately, I was in the hospital so long that they needed to keep inserting new PICCs throughout my arms and wrists. It always hurt.

Back to the important stuff. Food. Soon, my small shelf was overflowing with fruits, veggies, and "real treats." Then one day, Carol showed up with the perfect storage center: a mini-fridge. We moved a set of drawers to a spot near my recliner and put the fridge on it. I had an abundance of food and now we had a place to store my snacks. My friend, Charlie, asked me about my favorite fruit. Pineapple. After that, with each visit, he brought in a fresh cut up pineapple for our fruit center. I began to have such an abundance of food that, even with a fridge, we were beginning to have a storage-center problem.

But Carol brought in a knife, utterly against hospital rules, and after that, even a giant watermelon would have been fine for storage. Todd, on observing several of my meals, became concerned about the lack of what he considered "ample protein." This was not a guessing exercise for him. He is a fitness trainer with considerable education in dietetic issues. He began bringing in approved protein drinks. They were flavors I liked, so he knew I would drink them. And I did. I was hoping drinking them would give me six-pack abs. Apparently, it does not work that way.

A humorous byproduct of my room mini-fridge was the angst it caused for the nurses on the ward. Word got around there was one in my room. Other patients began to ask the nurses, and even the doctors, how to get theirs. One day, Carol was asked directly how she managed to get a mini-fridge into my room.

"I just brought it in."

Did I say Carol was born and raised in New York?

This might be as good a time as any to bring up one of the most important words I learned from my stay: "advocate." In my case, I had several. The most obvious was Carol Clews. I think we all know that by now. Carol was there day in and day out. Carol let nothing slide. Ashleigh was the second. They were bolstered by the nursing and tech staff. Even the housekeeping staff, whom I had grown to love, watched out for me. I cannot write of advocacy without acknowledging Dr. Feller. The nurses often told us that she was her patients' best advocate. "No one messes with Dr. Feller's patients." To wit: one day, Carol was visiting me when a usually pleasant nurse practitioner was in my room checking on me. I was asking her about some significant neuropathy pain I was experiencing in my feet. For some reason I will never understand, the nurse began to berate me.

"You don't know what real pain is. Wait till after the surgery. Your chest will be in unbelievable pain from having your sternum split open. Your ribs will be broken. And I'll tell you something else, Mr. Clews, if you have neuropathy, you just might be taken off the transplant list."

Until that very moment, this nurse had been wonderful. We could not believe our ears. It was devastating. It frightened Carol as much as anything we had heard since the diagnosis. And we had heard some pretty bad stuff. Carol suddenly left the room. She went downstairs and headed for the cafeteria to get a cup of coffee and try to calm herself. She later described what happened next.

"I was walking blindly, my world having been suddenly turned upside down. I wasn't seeing anything. I almost ran smack into Dr. Feller. She asked me right away what was wrong. I blurted out the whole incident. She looked me straight in the eye and said, 'Don't you give this another thought. I'm the only one you should listen to about Mr. Clews' transplant status.'"

Carol felt that her encounter with Dr. Feller was propitious, if not divine. I don't know what happened after that, but I never saw the nurse again. Folks, that is an advocate. Again, the insensitivity of that nurse was an anomaly. More typical of the nurses' empathy for their patients was the nurse with me one night, late in my stay, when I was in pain and felt defeated. As we talked, she broke down and cried. Remarkably, it was one I had often described as "flippant." I'll repeat: the nurses were angels.

# Chapter 17
# Get Naked

Aside from my neuropathy, my central body was holding its own. It turned out my brain, on the other hand, was losing its grip. Mentally, I began to weaken. All I wanted to do was sleep. My little walking slips of paper for keeping track of laps had become orphans. More critically, I became disoriented. My attempts at conversation made little sense. In other words, to all of those around me, nothing had changed. However, on one occasion when the nurses were unable to wake me, the doctors were called immediately. In response to my disorientation, I was taken for a brain scan. On my way, I decided to make sure they would find nothing embarrassing, so I did a mental sweep. The first thing I did was clear out those few sensuous thoughts I may have had about a nurse or so. And those I regularly had about Carol. Marital privacy, you know. My brain scan came back normal, much to the surprise of my whole family. In fact, they suggested a do-over. The doctors determined that the reason for my actions, and inactions, was that my sodium level had taken another critical drop. A message to any wife taking salt away from your husband: if he seems not to be making sense to you, immediately return his salt shaker. My sodium was increased in the form of a regular dose of liquid potassium. A small-portion cup of potassium drink. Sodium. Salt. Think of a cup of thick, liquid salt. I had never put anything that disgusting in my mouth, with the exception of something (and I still do not know what it was) gelatinous, with little black round things throughout it, I ate in Cambodia. I was given one cup of sodium with each meal. It worked. My potassium levels soon returned to normal. Healthy in mind, if not in body.

There was more good news. Dr. Feller informed us that the review committee had decided to extend my 1A status for three months. That was, again, one of those good news/bad news deals for me. My chances for a heart remained high. My possibilities for going home to wait were low. Being in the hospital helped me stay 1A. We all agreed, the best way to go home was with a new heart and a healthy body. Even my legs were responding to daily treatments to reduce the distress and soreness from the swelling. Kudos to Brent.

Once again, things seemed to be going in the right direction when, one morning, I noticed that my jaw hurt. I found out why when I began brushing my teeth. I touched a spot near the back of one side of my mouth. "Holy carrrumba! What the hell was that?" Sharp, intense pain shot through that area and right into the rest of my head. I touched it again. Yep, that was the spot. The last time I remembered that kind of pain was when my fingers decided to each do the individual walkabout. I looked in my mouth expecting to see a volcano in the back of my mouth. Nothing out of the ordinary. Still, that entire side of my head hurt. I went back to bed and called for a nurse. The upshot? I needed to have a tooth extracted. It was infected, and no infections were allowed in my room, let alone in my body.

There was a silver lining in all of this: the University of Maryland School of Dentistry is right on the same campus as the hospital. So I was carted directly there. I was introduced to a dental resident who looked inside my mouth and shot me up with Novocain. Then she left while it kicked in. I waited and waited for her to come back. From my perch, I could see her just down the hall, chatting it up with some friends. I waited some more. Now, we should establish that I am a dental coward. I agonize less about having surgery than I do about having my teeth cleaned. I began to fear the Novocain was wearing off. I tapped my teeth just to check. Yes, it was wearing off. I was sure of it. I finally got up and, in my hospital gown with an open back, and drooling down the front of my pretty dental bib, walked down the hall to the dentists' klatch.

"Excuse me, I don't want to be a party pooper, but are you going to wait until my oral opioid wears off completely to start working on my tooth? If that's your plan, they'll find me in the halls working my way back to my room."

I was pissed. She instructed me to go back to the chair, said there was plenty of time before the drug wore off and that she soon would be there. I walked back to my chair, probably inadvertently mooning both her and her friends. Shortly after that, she appeared and pulled the tooth. It hurt. I suspected that she had not yet had her classes in "Bedside Manner" and "Elements of Novocain." I spent the next several days in quite a bit of pain. Just one of those things, I guessed. No one was very happy about the episode, particularly my long-time dentist. After I returned home and subsequently visited him, I told the story. He was pretty unhappy about the whole situation. He said I should have called him to come and take care of it.

The funny thing is, he probably would have done it. Of note is that he went to Duke and, at that time, Maryland and Duke were huge basketball rivals. I am certain the episode only added to his distaste for his Maryland Terrapins rival.

Shortly after I healed from the tooth horror event, I had the best night I had had since I entered the hospital. Carol had spoken to the ward staff and asked if they could help arrange for a bed to be put in my room so she could spend the night with me. They pulled strings, probably ropes, and got the bed. *Wonderful*. Wait, that word is not good enough. But there is not one that would adequately describe my joy at the thought that Carol and I would be sleeping in the same room again. Even if it had to be in separate beds. By then, it had been well over a year since we had been in bed together, even slept in the same room. If Carol had to be in another bed, so be it. We were in the same room. As soon as we were alone, I pulled up my gown.

"Take all your clothes off. Get naked."

Well, what do you expect? I had a heart condition. I wasn't dead.

"Put that gown down or I'm leaving."

"Get naked or I'm leaving."

"Vince, I'm not kidding. Someone's going to walk in…put it down!"

"You're kidding?" Putting my gown down, but not giving up, I continued, "Come on. You're going to have to change anyway. Why not do it so I can watch?"

I wasn't kidding. Over a year or so prior to my becoming ill, the minister and I were having lunch. Great guy. Then in his early forties. Always a joy to be with. The two of us were sitting at a picnic table on the church grounds, eating our sandwiches.

"Vince, what do you love doing more than any other thing in the world?"

I think the answer was supposed to be, "Reading the Bible and praying."

"Watching Carol undress."

In a second, he was sprawled across the table, laughing. I love a man of the cloth who can enjoy the humor of reality. Although I suspect he will never again ask a parishioner that question.

Back at the hospital, Carol changed in the bathroom. She said it was because a nurse or tech might walk in and see her undressed.

"Lock them out."

Nothing I said worked. I moved over so there would be plenty of room for her in my bed when she came out. When she did, she was in pajamas. I admit to a little disappointment because I had left one of my clean, easy-access gowns especially for her. I patted her spot in the bed.

"All right, but just while we watch TV."

"I checked. They don't have those channels here."

Carol gave me one of those "You're an asshole" looks. She climbed into bed with me. How long had it been? We held each other. It was too emotional. Carol cried. As the man of the room, I felt it my duty to stay strong. But God, was I struggling. We finally settled and were holding each other. At one point, I thought I heard the door open. But who cared? The Pope could have walked in, and he could not have gotten a wafer between us. Carol stayed in the bed with me until we decided it was time to go to sleep. Then she got into her bed. The bad news: I wanted to roll over so I could watch her sleep, but I was holding just enough fluid and was weak enough that I was unable to make the move. I could not get off my back. I grabbed the bed rail and pulled myself over as much as I could so I could look at her beside me, even for just a few seconds.

"Good night, Carol. I love you."

"I love you, too. Just think, it won't be long before you'll be home with a new heart. And you'll be healthy, just like you were before. This will be over before we know it."

# Chapter 18
# A Lesson About Birds

My "Uncle Buck" look was addressed shortly after the overnight event. And it was a big success. I lost nearly forty-five pounds of fluid. Forty-five pounds in a few weeks. Now, where are my Speedos? Come on, there are people on TV bragging about losing fifteen pounds in eight weeks. I should have taken out a full page ad in *The Examiner*. "Lose more weight faster." The catch was that first you have to hold enough fluid to be dying.

The real key to extracting so much fluid so fast was time spent on a machine called a hemopurifier. It is a dialysis machine that routinely draws thin fibers to capture and remove viruses from the blood it filtered. The "purified" blood is then returned back into the body. In my case, the machine was not used to remove viruses. Rather, it removed water from the blood. Connecting the system to me required a procedure, aka surgery. This might be as good a time as any to address the word "procedure." In my case, the "procedure" required that the docs wheel me into an "operating" room (OR). Note: it was not called a "procedure" room. There is no PR. Here is the deal simplified: procedures are what happens to other people. What happens to you is always surgery.

I was returned to my room, where I had to spend the next several days attached to a smaller version of the hemopurifier. One day, still on the machine and simultaneously working on my computer, I moved to reach for something. My motion pulled the tube attached to the machine right out of me. Blood shot everywhere. I beeped for help. When the nurse walked in and saw what certainly must have looked like a bloodbath, she yelled for help. In a moment, I was surrounded by nurses and techs. One nurse, a big man, attempted to get to me but was blocked by the table. He grabbed it and pushed it out of the way. I pulled the table back to stop him from moving it because I had not had a chance to save what I was writing on the computer. He yelled for me to let go. I yelled back that I needed to save my work. Let's get perspective here. I was trying to save words. He was trying to save my life. I guess my attitude and struggle with him really aggravated him. He grabbed the table and flung it out of his way. I do not know what kept the computer on the table, but if it had hit a wall, no "transplant" would have saved my document. I decided he meant business and shut up. In short order, the nurses stopped the bleeding. By the time the crisis was resolved, there was blood everywhere. My sheets were soaked with blood. I was pretty well covered, too. The scene reminded me of being in old Miss Effie Ditto's backyard after she would twist the head off one of her chickens and it would flop around all over the yard, blood shooting hither and yon. As for my room, a wonderful tech began the cleanup, getting both my room and me cleaned and back into shipshape. God bless her. What a wonderful woman. Let me say it again: I had dear, caring techs throughout my entire stay. I was grateful for their work and enjoyed their company.

One, a young tech named Sean, was maybe in his early thirties. He always worked over-and-above his job and had a great sense of humor. He regularly spun a particular outrageous yarn with the nurses, especially any new ones. And he caught Carol in it. It was wonderful. He insisted that he had fourteen children, each by a different "momma." Carol was stunned.

"Yea, that's it. Fourteen children. All over the place."

"How do you keep track of all those birthdays?"

"I don't. Too many to track."

"I guess so." Carol was now in utter shock. "My, gosh…I mean, you must work more than one job. Surely you don't make enough here, I mean, to cover all that child support."

"I don't pay any child support."

"You don't pay any child support."

"Of course not. Why should I do that?"

"Well, they're your children. Certainly, you have some obligation to help the mothers…I mean, to—"

"No, ma'am. That's up to the mommas. They're the ones that had the babies."

"But they're your children!"

"No. You ain't seeing it. If those women did not want to have to support those babies, then they should not have had them. I ain't supporting no kid I did not have."

The disbelief then turned to ire. Carol just could not believe what she was hearing. After he took her to the point where I hid the fruit knife, he gave up the game. He was a happily married man with two adorable children. His humor was a great break from the drudgery of the stay. I loved watching him work people, especially my very gullible wife.

The bloody spectacle in my room had been resolved. But still not the fluid issue. My fluid was still fighting to hold onto territory it had gained, with headquarters now set up in my abdomen. Great. My belly was back. I looked like I was just short of delivery. I gained a whole new respect for pregnant women at thirty-four weeks. It reinforced my theory that God is a man. What Creator would ever give his own gender menstrual cycles, the discomfort of a baby belly, the pain of childbirth, and menopause? We men are tough, but obviously not tough enough for all of that. One day I found that out for certain. It was not just my stomach that swelled. The term "scrotum cozy" might suffice to explain. That you know even that much is because I won another one of those "It's *my* book" moments with Carol. The excessive bloating caused the doctors to do an abdominal ultrasound.

"Abdominal? Abdominal? The life-or-death battle is going on in the hills just south of there, Doc!"

They stuck with the abdomen. Whatever they found was not good because there was discussion about surgery.

"Okay, I'm with you. Let's stick with the abdomen."

Happily, the decision was made to waylay the surgery. Instead, they would keep draining the fluid, as well as reduce my fluid intake. Over the next week or so, I took in less fluid than a desert straggler. It was tough. My fluid intake was limited to things that looked like ear swabs with wetted tips. I would suck on the swab and rub the residual dampness on my lips. I was never "not thirsty." And I was still retaining fluid. That, of course, meant that my adrenal system was yelling, "Like hell I'm going to work!"

It was just about this time that what had been progressive healing on my legs took a turn in the opposite direction. Suddenly they were getting painful again, the result of "The Return of the Open Sores." It remained very painful each time the stockings were removed and put back on my torn skin. As the week wore on and the pain increased, I saw no reason why they should not just shoot me and end it. They would not, so I decided to do it myself...in a fashion. When patients are in continuously bad pain, sometimes they are given a little pump with a push button. Press the button, and it releases a prescribed amount of a painkiller into the system. I got a case of Tommy John thumb from pressing it so much. Apparently, we patients were not to be trusted. After the system gave the prescribed dose, any relief from continued pressing was imagined. Imagine that. Frankly, the prescribed dosage was not much help. Carol would sometimes gently touch one of my legs. Funny how she was being loving, and I was yelling for the nurses.

"Make her stop. Take her away. Even if you have to strap her down and roll her out. Get her away from my legs."

Pain, even soothed at the hands of someone you love, can never be an aphrodisiac. No one could figure out why the pain had returned. And at such an intense level. Of more concern was the infection potential, accompanied by the new eruptions. The issue was finally resolved, and the pain subsided, when Brent returned to the scene. He was shocked at the decline but soon resolved the matter. As I understood it, a substitute nurse, attempting to help, placed a different kind of medicated pads on the wounds. Each time the pads were removed, they pulled any healing away with them. I am sure it was more complicated than that, but we can go with that for the moment and move on. Once Brent began his work on my lower legs, they began to heal. The improvement seemed almost immediate. The sores that were the size of half a dollar began to decrease to smaller denominations. Reaching the quarter was a big deal for us. The nurses, the techs, and the housekeeping staff all cheered my shrinking-wound progress. One outcome of the sore episode was that I limited visits from people outside the family. The pain, and accompanying angst, was so bad that the thought of entertaining was beyond my capability. I also looked dreadful. I just did not want people to remember me "that way." As "that way" lingered, I suspect there was another lottery among the bettors on the ward. "Soreless legs day."

In time, my legs began to feel better, and I surfed toward normal. As normal as life can be when you are dying and the only way that can change is if someone you do not even know dies first. Who in the world ever thinks that he or she would be in a situation like that? As my legs were healing nicely, the infection decided to move some of its progeny to a new area. "Let's try his, his…mouth!" That's right. They set up camp in my mouth. The infection was called "*thrush*." Who gives a vile mouth infection the name of a sweet songbird? Infections are killers—at least for me they could be. I do not know why, but I did not wind up in the ICU for this one. Maybe because it was isolated and could be treated without a lot of high-potency drugs being pushed through my veins into my larger system. For reasons I did not know, but gladly accepted, the battle took place solely in my mouth. And it was treated there. With every meal, which I was in too much pain to eat, I was given a little cup of something vile that I was to rinse around in my mouth. I had to swish it for a minute. Then I had a choice—to spit it out or drink it. "Drink it!? I thought we were trying to kill the infection, not me." It was several unpleasant weeks before the infection was gone. I was not a fan of the food, but it sure was good to eat again without the attendant "fixings."

You know the old "when it rains, it pours" adage? It was pouring on me. No sooner was my mouth healed than I had to have another "procedure" so they could place a swan in my neck. That was the end of Carol kissing me. She hates birds. I have decided that I should provide a formal definition of this procedure because there should be no confusion about what happens. The website for the National Library of Medicine says the "Swan-Ganz catheterization is the passing of a thin tube (catheter) into the right side of the heart and the arteries leading to the heart and the arteries leading to the lungs. It is done to monitor the heart's function and blood flow and pressures in and around the heart." Now, get this last sentence in the definition: "This test is most often done on people who are very ill." That's right. Just keep piling it on. The whole incident was literally (this has to be said) a pain in the neck. The biggest problem for me was that this device I was now going to be connected to meant that, once again, I could not leave my bed. Again with the urinal and the bedpan. The swan stayed in for a week. Another procedure, and it was gone. The good news is that the docs liked the information it generated. I was as strong, they said, as anyone in my condition could be expected to be. I say we leave the bedpan matter alone and close this chapter on a positive note.

# Chapter 19
# Exactly Right

I was feeling better. Maybe it was just compared to all the issues I had been going through prior to that moment. Maybe I just believed the doctors and family when they told me I looked better. Maybe because my numbers on critical issues like sodium, fluid, and various pressures were more in line with where they should have been. Or maybe all the prayers were working. The fact was that I was feeling better.

You are waiting for the other green sock to drop, aren't you? For the moment, there was no incident. I felt good enough to enjoy visits from friends. Maybe that was because they usually came bearing gifts. One especially dear friend, Donna Faw, brought me a copy of the book *Unbroken*. For those unfamiliar with either the book or the movie, it is the Laura Hillenbrand biography of Louis Zamperini, a World War II American prisoner of war (POW). The book focused mostly on his time in Japanese POW camps. The vividly written details of the grueling years of beatings, starvation, and further kinds of inhumane mistreatment caused me to have nightmares. At one point, I put away the book for a dose of relief. One thing was for certain, reading it limited the number of pity parties I threw for myself.

As I continued to feel stronger and my legs were in less pain, we decided I should begin walking again. I picked up where I left off, following my ward circuit. I pulled out the now sacred little white slips of paper that I had used earlier to count my trips. My first trips were to the reception desk at the entrance to the ward. The receptionist was a gracious woman of strong faith who always had a word of encouragement. Between the fealty of the receptionist and Brent, if I had not known better, I would have thought I had been transferred to a Baptist hospital.

One day when Carol joined me for my walk time, as she often did, we decided it might be fun to take an elevator down to the lobby. Cautious Carol found a wheelchair, and with the blessings of the nurses, we took the three-floor elevator ride from the ward to the lobby. We found a bench, and Carol sat down with me. It felt so good to see civilians, to smell air that was not the stale odor of my sanitized room. One wonderful aroma that wafted our way was from the ovens of the nearby fresh-cookie stand. I basked in its oatmeal raisin bouquet. From that day forward, a trip to the lobby became a frequent part of Carol's visits. And so did the purchase of an occasional cookie. Carol was always dressed for work or leisure. I, on the other hand, probably looked a little like John Belushi's slovenly character in *Animal House*. I wore my two-gown special accessorized with my green socks. No underwear. Conversations on our lobby bench with Carol, and Ashleigh when she walked my wheelchair, were checkered with "Don't sit like that," or "Pull your gown down."

Occasionally, I had visitors who found out that the guy they had always known as Vince Clews was not a patient at the hospital. Nor was Vincent Clews. On anything formal, I am William Clews. Few people know that that is even one of my names. To all my friends I am Vince. In no time, we had "a failure to communicate."

"I'm here to see Vince Clews."

"Hmmmm, we don't have a Vince Clews here."

"Are you sure? I'm pretty certain he's at this hospital.

"I don't see a Vince or Vincent Clews here."

The name issue caused a few of my acquaintances to leave without a visit. Ultimately, I was there long enough for my friends to know which name to ask for.

"I'm here to see William Clews."

"Oh, you mean Vince."

I never met most of the people at the front desk, but Carol, as well as other visitors, always described them as "the nice people at the front desk."

Just because a visitor got past them and to my room did not mean that we spent time together. Published patient schedules are not necessarily the prescribed one on a given day. The visitor who was waved through sometimes would come to my room, only to find out that I was gone for several hours.

"Oh, I'm so sorry. Mr. Clews is not here right now."

"Oh. He said he had a clear day, to come on down. Do you know when he'll be back?"

"I can't be specific, but it's going to be a while. Would you like to leave a note?"

Most people would do that. Some found ways to kill time and came back later. Too often visitors would come to see me, and the reward for their effort was unrewarding, to say the least. The longer I was there, the more apt it was to happen.

"Hi, Vince. Carol said it would be okay if we stopped in for a few minutes just to say hello."

"Gosh, it's great to see you. How're you doing?"

"We're fine. You look so good."

"Thanks. I'm feeling great. A couple of days ago, they...zzzzzzz."

That visit must have been a real rewarding experience. Between exhaustion and drugs, I was seldom able to make it through a whole day without a nap. Or two. And I never knew when that would happen. One time when Chris was coming to town, Ashleigh got the two of them tickets for an Orioles game. Box seats. On the way to the game, they stopped by for a surprise visit. I was thrilled to see them, especially Chris, as I seldom saw him. I had the pregame show on. We talked so long, the game started. I told them to get going. But they decided to watch the game with me. That sounded great to me. Watching the game with my kids. Of course, I fell asleep. When I awoke, several innings later, the nurse said that she told them to leave. Good. I could well have slept through all the remaining innings. Some fan. I actually called the kids and asked them to come back and watch the rest of the game with me. Some father. And they did. Some children.

I was now just over two months in the hospital. In fact, on September 5, I spent my seventieth birthday there. Carol brought in cards and placed them around the room. I got some special gifts. One was from a four-year-old boy, Austin, whose military parents were friends of Chris. It was a big yellow banner with the outline of outstretched arms on it. He had been told about me and wanted to give me a hug. "The banner (which now hangs in my office) worked just fine, Austin." There was also a handwritten note from four-year-old Hank. Before I went in the hospital he made me cookies, which we ate together. He was a little fellow who, on Sunday mornings, would walk up to the end of a pew where I was sitting. He would stand there for a minute or so and just stare at me with great concern. "I'm fine now, Hank." My then very young granddaughter, Kailey, (to whom I am Nonno) gave me drawings of the sun to remind me things would get better. "Those were the gems in the room, honey." One gift I received on that birthday day was a special honor. It was a cup with a big numeral 5 (for the $5^{th}$) on it. The nurses gave it to me. My biggest gift was that I was pretty much pain-free. Oh yeah, and alive.

The surgical procedures had settled down to a precious few. My routines, unless otherwise interrupted, were pretty consistent. Blood draws in the morning and, usually, once or twice more during the day. Walks. Watching TV. I became a regular viewer of *Duck Dynasty*. My brother Carter was a huge fan and got me hooked on the show and the Dynasty books.

Baseball season was drawing to a close, and the Orioles were in the hunt for the playoffs. In the evening, I would get into my recliner, settle in with a snack, and watch that evening's game. Carol brought me some bouillon squares. I would order (I make it sound like room service)—let me start over. I would *request* some hot water and have a chicken-flavored drink with crackers. If it was a warm evening, instead of bouillon I would grab a drink from my little fridge. "Livin' the life." Except for this: I was not "livin' it" with Carol. Her absence was particularly tough during specific time blocks. One was dinner time or, if you are a Southerner, suppertime. Her regular routine was to come to see me after work, which meant that she would get to my room around the time they served dinner. As the clock moved toward 5:00, I would become anxious. I knew she would not be there at 5:00. Generally, though, that meant she had left the office and was on her way. I would begin to think only about her imminent arrival. I had not been home for nearly three months. The absence was getting tough. I craved her presence. When she walked into the room, it became home.

The other rough time in the visit framework was weekend mornings. They were killers. I would be awakened between 5:00 and 6:00, just as if it were a weekday. Then the wait time began. I knew Carol was coming earlier on those days. I wanted her there as early as possible so we could spend the full day together. But Saturdays were her only day to sleep past 5:00 a.m. She more than earned that privilege. It was also her only full day to run errands, clean the house, and so on and so on. They were all things she had to do. We would talk as early as possible, and she would estimate a time that she thought she could arrive. Hell, she may as well have stamped that estimate right on my eyeballs. That was all I could see. I was experiencing the "loneliness of the long-distance married transplant patient." Sunday mornings were tough, too. Carol was committed to her faith and the support she found in community worship. She bathed in the loving prayer and provision of our pastor and fellow congregants. At the same time, there was the other side of Sunday mornings—the great desire to be with me for as long as she could on this work-free day. A kind of Desdemona, "I do perceive here a divided duty" situation. I knew where I stood on the where-to-be issue and was often vocal about it. In retrospect, as much as I tried to show patience about my anxiety to see her, I was utterly selfish.

I got her undivided attention one afternoon when she came in after work and my arms were pretty heavily bandaged. I also had a few bandages here and there at points over the rest of my body. And I was moving very gingerly, when I moved at all.

"What happened to your arms?"

We all know how there are things we sure wish we could keep from someone we love because we know that when that person finds out, she is going to be all over us like a rash.

"I banged them on the walls."

"The walls? How did you bang them on the walls?"

I knew I was too far in.

"Last night I got out of bed and kind of stumbled."

"My God, what happened?"

"I had to take a leak, and I thought there was a urinal on the other side of my bed, so I was walking around to it..."

"A urinal? There's no urinal in this room."

"Yeah. I know that now. Somehow it made sense then."

"So what does a supposed 'urinal in the room' have to do with the bandages?"

"Well, on the way around the bed, I began to stumble against the walls …"

"What? Why were you stumbling? What do you mean, 'stumble against the walls'?"

"Just stumble. I guess I cut my arms banging into the wall. The next thing I knew, I was on the floor. I don't remember anything after that."

In fact, until they cleaned them, the walls looked like my room had been the location for a recreation of the St. Valentine's Day Massacre. At some point in my narrative, a nurse came in. She finished describing the episode.

"Hi, Mrs. Clews. Mr. Clews is going to be fine. He apparently stumbled around until he finally fell. We had no idea what was going on. Honestly, it was fortunate that someone came to do his vitals. We found him sitting on the floor in a pool of blood."

"What? A pool?"

"Yes. I'm sorry. We had no idea he was up or had fallen. If he yelled, we didn't hear it. It's just so fortunate that we found him. He lost so much blood."

"You mean he could have bled out right there on the floor."

"Thank God, we found him in time."

I felt we could use some levity, so I chimed in.

"Let's look at the positive side of things, honey. If I had bled out, it would have saved you money on the embalming."

I was the only one who thought that was funny. That seemed to be a constant on my transplant journey. In fact, I had lost a lot of blood. And, I do remember sitting surrounded by a bloody floor. After that event, the rails on my bed were kept up, especially at night. Just like a crib. And some kind of alarm system was initiated that caused a noise if I tried to get out of the bed. That seemed to me to be adding insult to injury. As for enduring reminders of hitting the wall, I still have multiple scarred areas on my forearms where the skin was torn away. Those spots are still pretty sensitive, too. And they still bleed when I bang hard into a wall. I try not to do that in other people's homes.

The wait for a heart was beginning to wear on me. "Someone with a matching heart out there somewhere must have 'shed this mortal coil.'" At that time, through my brother, I had made the acquaintance of a retired hit man. I know this is going to sound crazy, but he was a very nice guy. Carter, who had introduced me to him, would always tell me, "T (What do you think—I'm going to put his name here?) asked about you and sends his regards." I always wanted to suggest to Carter that he ask T if he could help find me a heart...if you know what I mean. Back in the real world, I knew that the doctors were doing all that they could to stay on top of the available heart market, so I was always reluctant to ask Dr. Feller about the progress. However, one time when Carol was visiting, I thought I would ask the doctor the question on both of our minds.

"How's the hunt going?"

She said she was receiving calls pretty consistently about potential matches. But, she insisted, she had not found that one that was exactly right. And, she further added, she was not accepting anything short of "exactly right." I thought, as the patient waiting for a heart that "right" was close enough. Years later, as the patient alive, healthy, and writing this book, I appreciate "exactly right."

While I was waiting for my "exactly right" heart, the Orioles broke my old one. As the season was ending, so was their run for the playoffs. I tried to believe that they did not know what they were doing to me. The good news was that football season had started, so my focus quickly shifted to the Ravens, our pro football team. A new Sunday routine set in. Carol still would go to the early service at church, then pick up the newspaper and come to spend the afternoon. No change there. But shortly before the one o'clock kickoff time, "the group" would start pouring in. The "group" was the same one that always came to our house for the games. Mike, Ashleigh, Carter and, on rare occasions when he was in town, Chris. We would all gather around the TV, watch the game and eat snacks provided by Carol, who had no interest in football whatsoever. We would yell and, after every poor play, take turns throwing my Ravens purple foam brick at the screen. The hospital afternoons required only two changes for us from our home stadium: crowding around a smaller screen and "no yelling." An occasional reminder from Carol was required to keep us, especially Mike, quiet. Sunday visits by Carol during football season were a special sign of her love for me.

I tried hard to show her my appreciation by giving her my attention during time-outs.

It was during this season in my stay that I had a unique experience. Maryland Public Television (MPT), where I had developed the CSK series, decided to initiate a Wall of Fame to honor selected employees. I was one of the people being honored. Need I say that I was unable to attend the event? So why does this story matter? UMMC worked with the people at MPT, particularly Fran Minakowski and George Beneman, to provide a live feed of the activities to my room. Miles and miles away from the event, Carol and I, thanks to my former employer and the hospital, sat in my room and watched the ceremony. That is what I call patient services. MPT also arranged for the ceremonies to be put on a DVD so I could view them later, just in case I slept through the event.

My physical well-being was in a peculiar place at this point in the wait for the transplant. My heart was getting worse as time was passing. My overall health was deteriorating, too. But, as I indicated earlier, life was good. How is that for an oxymoron? However, my kidneys were still working. My sodium levels were acceptable. My weight was again dropping, a reflection of fluid passing through my system with minimal problems. I was 1A. Top of the list for a heart. Carol and I continued our walks to the lobby, and I had an occasional cookie. Well, every time we were near the bakery, I had one. By now I was wearing my bathrobe and slippers. I had only changed over to the slippers after the assurance by Carol that she would take my green socks home, wash them, and put them in a secure place where she could get them back to me if I ever backslid from my slippers into socks again. One day when the weather was that really "autumn nice," we expanded our walk to venture out onto the sidewalk. Soon we were walking (well, I was being wheelchaired) onto the sidewalk along the front of the hospital. I could feel an occasional gentle breeze. Air that was moving. It was hard to believe something so common could feel so good. I took deep breaths, primarily inhaling exhaust fumes. That was fine. Anything that smelled different than my stale room and medication worked for me. Breezes, odors, and a sense of freedom. I was finally the guy on the sidewalk that I so often saw from my window.

My visits beyond the walls of the hospital became a once- or twice-a-week treat. Sometimes my "walk" was with Carol, other times with Ashleigh, and occasionally with both. One day, we actually crossed the street to the small park, found a bench, and sat for a while. The journey from my room to the park became a semi-regular part of visits. Occasionally I would look at the building, specifically at what I was sure was my window. I could see myself leaning on the sill, longingly watching the passers-by. Every time we would go to the park, we would pass a hot-dog vendor. When I used to watch people going to ball games and see them buy a hot dog from that guy, I wanted one. A hot dog on your plate is not the same as a hot dog from a vendor. I spent one college summer working in a room where we prepared "dogs" and drinks for the vendors to sell to the fans. Vendor dogs are special. For one thing, the hot dog on your plate does not have the hint of a bin of old, greasy water. I really wanted a vendor hot dog. "Touch of mustard, catsup, and lots of chili on top, please." Carol was adamant that there would be no vendor dog for me. "Bacteria, infection, sepsis, death." We enjoyed wonderful times in the park, sans hot dog. I settled for being thankful to be with Carol outside, looking in.

# Chapter 20
# Chopped Beef Patties Are Flat

Inside, my room was going through a bit of a metamorphosis. Okay, that may be an overstatement. But it had become less the *room assigned to me* and more *my room*. I had now been in it long enough for it to have become pretty personalized. There were, of course, get-well cards placed around the room. Carol brought them in for me to see and then took most home because there was a "no tape or pushpin on the walls" policy. Still, the corner with my recliner, my fridge, my food bin, my slippers, and my robe hanging on an adjacent wall added to the sense of ownership of the room. There were nurses who cared for my health needs, techs who saw to it that, among other things far more important, my bed had fresh sheets and pillowcases every day. There was a housekeeping crew who made sure my room was clean and smelled good. And here was the kicker: all of them were kind, concerned, and became my hospital friends. I never lacked for good company.

I had another group of "friends" I saw almost every day. They were the regular hosts on The Food Network: *The Barefoot Contessa,* Jacques Pepin, Paula Deen, Giada (especially when she wore low-cut tops), and *The Great Food Truck Race*. I never missed *Chopped*. Ashleigh watched it at home, and we often talked about the episodes and who won. So here I was in the hospital, eating uninspiring food while I watched chefs making food to kill for. That was helpful.

One interesting aside. When I got home, for some reason, I stopped watching *Chopped*. In a conversation with Ash sometime later, I found out that, just about the same time, she had also stopped watching the show. I don't understand these things. I just write about them.

Because I was finally well enough to smile, friends and family sought ways to make my now becoming-extended hospital stay as good as it gets. Food often did the trick. Outside food, that is. For example, my buddy, Steve Yeager, brought me a dozen of my favorite: breaded and deep-fat-fried chicken gizzards from the famous Lexington Market. But the biggie was when Carol's organization had a crab feast. In Maryland, that means steamed crabs with Old Bay Seasoning, corn on the cob, slaw, and beer. That's enough to make any event a feast. During this stay, I missed that time of summer when cookouts and crab feasts were what eaters like me lived for. The day of her event, Carol said she would come to see me as soon as she could get away. And, of course, she did. With the nurses' permission, she came bearing gifts of crabs and corn on the cob. And near beer. The caution was that the seasoning had to be removed from the crabs before I could eat them. But there they were. Half a dozen crabs spread out in front of me on my bedside table. All mine. One does not eat crabs. One savors them. And then smells them for days on everything in the room. My room smelled a little like rancid seafood for a while. I am certain other patients were thinking, "If this whole thing doesn't work out, I sure hope I'm a better-smelling corpse than the guy in room sixty-three."

Our dear friend, Dedi, who was at her summer home in Maine, thrilled me and somehow escaped wrath when she had a same-day fresh lobster sent down for me. Imagine, I was sitting in a hospital bed in Baltimore eating freshly caught Maine lobster. Even the ordinarily generous-minded Dr. Feller was a little disturbed with the abundance of unapproved food I was being given. Shortly after Ashleigh and Chris brought me several more crabs, Ashleigh told me the good doctor let them know in no uncertain terms that I was to eat only approved foods. Still, I was so often the beneficiary of special food kindnesses of the "do not eat" sort, I still smile at the memories.

Sadly, the hospital food did not make me smile. There were times I just would not eat it. And I was pretty vocal about it. The problem was that anyone who would listen to my diatribes could do nothing about them. Carol was great about bringing me leftovers. Often, she would make something special, and approved, for me. The nurses generously let her use the staff microwave and refrigerator. Ashleigh also had to listen to me complain about missing foods I liked, such as pot pie. So she found a place that made low-salt, high-protein meals, and she would bring me a pot pie every so often. She even brought the menu so I could call in an order for her to pick up. Carol and Ashleigh were terrific about supplementing my hospital diet. Friends continued to send in food. We have a friend named Jeanne, a great cook and baker. She sent in everything from homemade *Bolognese* to lemon scones. The outside-supplied meals came to about half a dozen on a good week.

Other than those treats, I was still eating food I felt was lacking in flavor. One day, I decided it was time to take matters into my own hands. I used my cell phone to get the phone number for the administrative offices. I called and asked to speak to the administrative assistant to the Hospital Director.

An aside: When I began selling myself as a freelance writer, and then when I formed a company, I had a primary rule about meeting with a prospective client. If there is a second person in the room (I'm sorry if this is perceived as sexist), especially if it was a woman, give that person as much attention as, if not more than, you give the prospect. "Because," I would say to my salespeople, "you can be certain that when you leave, the prospect will turn to the other person and ask, 'What do you think about that (person, idea, pitch, etc.)?'" And, that answer would be the one that would count most in the decision maker's evaluation. So I made my call to the person I knew could most help move forward our conversation about the food.

"Hello. My name is William Clews."

"Yes, Mr. Clews?"

"I'm a patient in the hospital. I'm calling to discuss the quality of the food we are being served."

"Well, I'm afraid there's no one here who can help you right at the moment."

"That's fine. I'd be happy to talk with you, if you can give me a couple minutes."

"Sure. How can I help you?"

I described my food concerns with her, certain my remarks would go further than that conversation. I was right. Later that morning, a nice woman from the dietary office visited me. She may have headed the office. We talked about my concerns. She said something to the effect that she would pass them along. She left, and I fell asleep. That afternoon, she returned with several other staff members. She introduced them, including the man in the white double-breasted jacket. Only the toque was missing. The chef was in my room. I silently vowed not to fall asleep. He introduced himself and then the other people, who were all associated with food services. We talked about my issues with the food. It was a gentle sparring match that went something like this.

"Everything is bland."

"We can't season the food because we are serving more than three thousand patients. Their dietary limitations and reactions to foods vary widely. The safest procedure is to season nothing. As for your specific foods, you are allowed no salt. You are also allergic to lactose so, for instance, the pudding is lactose-free."

I was impressed. Still, I countered.

"There's no variety. I feel like I'm eating the same meal over and over."

"To a degree you are, Mr. Clews. We are a state institution working on a state budget. To meet the budget, we have to order in bulk. So we plan our meals on a four-day cycle."

A nice guy would have been very grateful for the special effort being made to accommodate his concerns. He might have said, "So nice of you to make this special trip. I understand. Thank you." Evidently not me.

"What's called a 'chopped beef patty' is round like a ball. I mean, it doesn't change the flavor, but it just doesn't look right. It is supposed to be flat."

"We serve it that way because it is fresh beef. It's more time efficient to scoop than it is to flatten it for each serving."

The man had viable answers for those questions and the others I brought up. He did say that he made up the menus, but the cooking is left to others. I made some crack about their day jobs being short-order cooks at local bars. I immediately had visions of him telling them what I said and them spitting in my food.

"My real point," I explained, "is that being in a hospital is completely demoralizing. There is little to look forward to on any given day, at any given moment. Meals should not fit into that category. They should be that one thing that is different. The thing you do look forward to. That's all I was trying to say. Make meals special."

The conversation wrapped up cordially, even friendly. They were nice people under a lot of pressure. Seems like a ubiquitous definition of hospital workers.

The next morning, my breakfast was served on a tray covered with linen. I even got a linen napkin. My plate was covered with a warmer, and the food was beautifully presented. My coffee was in a china cup. It looked like room service in a nice hotel. Lunch was the same, and so was dinner. This is a big deal. I was not getting the standard hospital fare. My over-easy eggs were actually over-easy, and warm. My noon sandwich looked like the delicious one you are shown in the fast-food ads but you never get when you go there. At dinner, my pork chop was thick and juicy. The nurses and techs called me names like "your Highness" and kissed my hand before they took my vitals. Carol was blown away. I think Ashleigh was embarrassed. I was delighted. The individual, and special, treatment continued for several days. I asked to see the chef. He came and, again, with his associates.

"Thank you for the wonderful food, the linens, the special forks, and all that. But I think I did not make myself clear. I wasn't asking for better treatment and food for just me. I was speaking for everyone. We should all be treated the same way."

It turned out he understood. Everyone should be treated the same way. My next meal was served on the tray with the old, ordinary utensils, and my coffee came in a Styrofoam cup. Oh, and there were no linens. It seems the part of the message that resonated on that second visit was that I was not asking for special treatment. Consequently, I never got it again. Dumb, dumb, dumb.

Before I leave the food aspect of my story, I have to mention the people who delivered the food to the rooms. A very few just walked in, slid the tray onto the table, and left. Most of them were as nice as they could be. They helped keep the bright days bright and brightened others. Wrong meal? They were on it. No creamer for the coffee? They found some. The only thing they could not do was make the pancakes warm again. And I'm certain, if they could have, they would have.

Physically, I was feeling pretty good for a dying man whose beard was now stark white and whose hair was turning gray. There were aspects of my health that did not always go so well. But nothing like the pain that I had suffered earlier. After almost three months of waiting, however, I was feeling a small crack in my stoicism. Where were all the hearts? I knew the doctors were staying on top of the search. Dr. Feller told us that there were several times when she thought she had one, but the heart was not "exactly right." She was holding up her end of the bargain. For the most part, I was, too. I walked every day. On good days, I added laps.

Carol and I increased our park visits. Interestingly, even with the number of vagrants who hung there, we never had a problem finding an empty bench. My feeling was that the brothers in the park made that happen because they felt warmly about the pretty young woman who was so faithful about visiting her old, dying father.

# Chapter 21
# A Day at the Races

There was a nurse who annoyed me. Carol thought she was delightful. I liked her but could have done without the histrionics and flawed attempts at humor. I have never been comfortable around over-the-top people. I know plenty of really funny professional entertainers. Comic actors, comedians, comediennes. They all have a sense of timing, know when they have hit the punchline, and stop. Know when to be funny and when not to. They are comics, not clowns. Big difference. The people I know who try to be funny seldom are. Funny, huh?

One day that particular nurse came in with a great idea. Baltimore was going to host its first, and probably only, Formula One Grand Prix race. That meant high-speed racing through the streets of the city, only this time with professional drivers. She decided getting out on a corner to watch the races was just what my tired heart needed. So I put on my trusty slippers and robe, and off we went. The nurse, Carol, and I in my wheelchair hustled down the elevators, out of the hospital, and across parking lots and down streets until we settled on a corner to wait for the race to begin. We waited and we waited. Nothing. We were just beginning to wonder, when ...*varooom, varooom, varooom*. There they came around the corner and right at us—and just as quickly, *varoom*!, they were gone. Thank God I was wearing my bathrobe. The way the wind hit us, had I not been wearing a tied-down robe, my gown would have been covering my head. Perhaps even been blown off. The race cars were speeding toward us, we could hear the roaring sound of the engines in our ears, and feel the wind as it swept by us—it was thrilling. I had not seen Carol that excited about anything non-cardiac-related in quite a while. I was pretty jacked, too. We stayed for maybe twenty minutes or so and headed back, chattering about the race the whole way to the hospital. On our return, the nurse noted that soon there would be Columbus Day fireworks in the Inner Harbor. She knew a great spot on the hospital roof where we would have a clear view. She said she would get me up there to watch them. The way her energy affected me was palpable. Carol was pretty popped, too.

The fireworks viewing never happened. Apparently, my ride to the races got back to a supervising nurse who was not buying it. "Our" nurse told us she had gotten some grief about the trip to the races. There would be no ride to the roof. Later that day, the supervising nurse—the one who blocked the pyrotechnics watch—came into my room. I expressed my indignation about her overbearing oversight. That was a mistake. Apparently Ashleigh was there. She subsequently took great delight in repeatedly telling the story of the nurse's response. In medical terms, she went through me like a saltwater enema. She said there would be no trip to watch the fireworks. Nor was I to go to the park anymore. In fact, I was not to leave the ward again. My unreceptive attitude to her edicts prompted her to become explicit about the rationale for adhering to her mandate.

"Every time you leave this ward, you drop to the bottom of the waiting list. You are no longer 1A. The right heart could become available, but you would not be the top recipient anymore because you were absent. The next in line would get it, and you would return to the bottom of the list."

Well, I guess I could see where that would be an issue. Nonetheless, I did not like the messenger. When I told Carol what the nurse had said, mimicking her voice, she did not see the nurse as a problem, not at all. She heard a thoughtful caretaker who was concerned about her patient. The supervisor implemented the change. I had had my last outing to the park. There would be no more trips, not even to the lobby. I was never going to have the up-against-the-glass smell of those fresh-baking oatmeal raisin cookies again. I was really angry with the nurse for her edict. Carol reminded me about my comment to her when she was so furious with the young Hopkins doctor she heard say that I was going to die.

"The messenger did not necessarily write the message." Her point was that it was Dr. Feller who put the limitations on my walks. So the next time I saw the good doctor, I asked her if that was true.

"The nurse is right. You need to be where you can be found on a moment's notice."

She did allow that I could go to the cookie area but that the nurses were always to know where I was. However, the trips to the park, and beyond, definitely were over.

# Chapter 22
# Sepsis, Sepsis

It was not long before my daily walks through the ward were changing. I was losing my strength. One by one, the slips of paper I carried with me for my count were being left behind in my room. "Hey, wait. What about me? We've been through it all for so long. To ward and hall and back. Is this how it all ends? A sliver of paper left on the scrapheap of history?" Based on my green-sock affection, you have certainly guessed by now that I kept all the slips. I felt I had to just in case my college ever decided to honor me. Surely they will want my "walking slips" on display. For now, however, what had originally begun as brisk marches around the ward and outside hall were becoming shuffles from my room to the receptionist desk and back. It was discouraging, so terribly discouraging.

It was at times like this that encouragement came from multiple sources. One, of course, was the community of friends who encouraged my faith, which at times went slip-sliding away. I felt increasingly like Job. "What is my strength that I should wait? And what is my end, that I should be patient?" On one visit from Fr. David, I told him I was discouraged and angry. It was hard for me, and sometimes Carol, to keep our heads above water and our hearts beneath the cross. I had had it. I was angry with everything, and that included God for putting us in this mess.

"Well, I think that's understandable. I think anyone in this situation would be upset."

"This has disrupted my whole life. It's killing Carol. I'm not just upset. I'm angry. I'm particularly angry at God."

"Of course you're angry. As for your anger at God, He's big enough to handle it. But you need to settle that with him. Let's pray about that right now."

On his next visit, David brought a selection of paper strips with Scripture verses on them he thought might help sustain my spiritual strength even as my physical strength waned. One of the passages read, "Be strong and courageous. Do not fear or be in dread of them, for it is the LORD your God who goes with you. He will not leave you or forsake you" (Deut. 31:6, ESV). Some days, they would help. Other days, I would not even finish reading the verse. Steve Floyd, a friend, and former client, sent me a card with a message of encouragement and, under his name, he had written "James 1:2-3." I had to look it up:

> Consider it pure joy, my brothers and sisters, whenever you face trials of many kinds, because you know that the testing of your faith produces perseverance. Let perseverance finish its work so that you may be mature and complete, not lacking anything.

It is amazing how many Bible passages encourage the weak to stay strong during rough times because it is part of a plan. For some reason, it reads well but can be a little grating when someone says it. I thought it was too easy to say that pain and struggle are part of God's plan when you are standing at the end of the bed instead of lying in it. Of course, there are too many stories of great works by those who recovered from the edge of death not to believe James's words or to dismiss my friends' encouragement. Nonetheless, boy, was I pissed off a lot.

There were times, however, when I made peace with my situation. It was during one of those times when, all of a sudden, it changed. I began to feel unwell. Sluggish. A complete lack of energy. Carol and Ash were visiting when a doctor on rounds stopped in to see me. He asked me a few questions, which I answered with questionable zest. Or not at all, according to my guests. Finally, he held up his fingers, changing the number of digits as he asked me to tell him how many I saw. I had no idea and, therefore, answered with the wrong number each time. Then he asked me to simply follow his finger as he moved it. I did not see any finger, moving or not. My effort to speak was slurred, and I was sliding into an unscheduled siesta. Suddenly, there was a burst of activity. I remember hearing one sentence: "Nurse, this man is septic. He's dying. Get him to the ICU *now*."

Typically, when patients are moved from area to area around the hospital, the activity is the responsibility of the transportation team. This time there was no call for transportation. Nurses and techs, even the doctor, all grabbed the bed, and I was out of there. Next stop, the ICU. My oxygen levels were low, and I was having trouble breathing. I could hear the Grim Reaper's scythe blow by my ear. The life-saver, Dr. Brian Barr, had me sedated and put on a ventilator. He ordered the swan reinserted and called for a central venous catheter (CVC), also called a "line." I tried to find a definition that most closely explained the CVC procedure. The following is from a blog called mighty-well.com. "It (the line) is also used for hyperalimentation, administering long-term IV therapy and drawing blood samples. The process involves the doctor cutting the skin near the collarbone. An anesthetic is given to numb the area. The doctor then threads the line's tip into a large vein above your heart. Meanwhile, the other end of the line is tunneled under the skin. It comes out of your chest. To keep it secure, the doctor puts in a stitch."

So there I was. On a ventilator with a tube sticking out of my mouth and a swan on my shoulder. And out for the count…thank God.

The sepsis situation was compounded (as if sepsis needs to be worse than it is) when the doctors could not find the source of the infection. And I was sinking. They used a broad spectrum of antibiotics to try to bring the infection and, in turn, the sepsis under control. The crisis continued well into the night. My life, once again, was hanging in the balance. Carol and Ashleigh were encouraged to spend the night. They were way ahead of the doctors in that regard. If the doctors had known the two warriors' record on "being there," they would have known that no request was required. They spent the night trying to sleep, through mental and emotional angst, on hospital furniture that routinely made sleeping a challenge. I, of course, was once again out of it, not knowing the crisis they were living through. In retrospect, I try to imagine what they went through at those times. I cannot. I think our imagination cannot conceive the strength it takes to survive the uncertainty during hours like that.

I did not die. I know you know that, but I love writing it. I awoke with Carol holding one hand and Ashleigh holding the other. I squeezed their hands. "Yep, I'm still here." A second one. "I love you." I was still heavily sedated, but clear on my messaging. The messages ended as I fell back into a heavy sleep. That was good. Real good, it turns out. When I awoke the next time, I realized something was in my mouth. Something was keeping me from moving it, at all. It was stuck open. My mouth would not close, so I could not swallow. You would be surprised how much anxiety that creates. My mouth was being held open wide, and, try as I may, I could not close it. I could not move it one iota. I felt terror. "What's going on? What's in my mouth?" I tried to bring my hand up to remove the offending obstacle, but I could not move my arm. Not at all. I tried my other arm. Stuck. I could not move it, either. I felt even more panicked. I need to remind you about my claustrophobia. If I feel I cannot move any single part of my body, in a very short time I cannot breathe. I know it sounds nuts, but I am a nutcase about claustrophobia. A ventilator is a claustrophobic's nightmare. I was on one. It is a machine that helps a patient who is unable to breathe on his or her own get air into the lungs. Everybody needs to breathe. The mouthpiece that held my mouth open was there so the tube from the ventilator could get air into my lungs so I could stay alive. But not move. I became hysterical. I did not give a damn what the people who put it in my mouth thought it was going to do. It was killing me. "Carol," I kept trying to mouth, "Help me. Help me. Help me." Ashleigh, Carol, and the nurses were trying to tell me to breathe through my nose. I was too petrified with fear to hear them.

"Breathe through your nose. Vince, listen. Breathe through your nose."

"Dad, you're okay. Just breathe through your nose. Dad, listen to Carol. Breathe through your nose."

I can now tell you something we all should know. If you have ever tried to hold down a pet while you were doing something for its own good while all it cared about was getting away, your soothing explanations did not mean squat to that guy.

I do not know how long it took for the message to get through to this frightened "pet," but to me it seemed an eternity. Finally, though, I tried nasal breathing. It worked. I was going to live. I could breathe. I kept pulling air through my large nose as fast as I could. You know the movies where guys like Jimmy Stewart played a cowboy lost in the desert, frantically looking for water. Then he suddenly finds it and cannot get enough. Call me cowboy.

A night of solid sleep with that thing in my mouth must have been the result of some mighty potent drugs. The infection, however, was still in my system, which meant I would be staying in ICU until it was under control. The big complication was continuing uncertainty about the exact source of the infection. That meant, of course, that there were still questions about how to treat it. My suggestion would have been a nice bowl of spaghetti and meat-a-balls, as my Aunt Margaret used to call them. That was not going to happen. I was intubated and, gratefully, kept pretty much out of it.

All the questions about cause and treatment finally came down to one for my family: "Is he going to make it?" A visit from Dr. Feller provided the answer. She told Carol and Ashleigh that my numbers were headed in the right direction and that she was happy with the way I was responding to the medication they had settled on using. She also promised to get me off the ventilator as quickly as possible. Once again, she was the bearer of good news. Spirits were lifted. I was able to comprehend just enough to muster a ventilator smile. Life still was not good on the device. But, by the end of the day, indications were that I was going to live to see another one…and many more. For the moment, that was good enough.

Oh yes, there was also this. In spite of my situation, which could have gotten me taken right off the list for a heart transplant, Dr. Feller told us she was going to make certain I stayed on it.

*"The good physician treats the disease. The great physician treats the patient who has the disease."- William Osler, Co-founder, Johns Hopkins Hospital*

# Chapter 23
# Up My Nose with a Ten-Foot Hose

It gets boring, doesn't it? The chapters keep opening with me still around. I have to say, however, I was getting a little tired of standing on the "Welcome" mat at death's door.

I began to accept the ventilator. That is, as much as I could accept having my mouth forced open 24/7. The pressure the aperture created on my jaws spawned another problem. Pain. I regularly would press my teeth down on the mouth monster and hold the position for as long as I could to relieve the pressure caused by my jaws being held wide open. Even just a second of relief from the constancy of the position would bring incredible relief. When I finally began to breathe through my nose with some consistency, they loosened my hands. The urge to reach up and pull out the mouthpiece was always there, but not so much that I would actually try it. At night, when instincts are more apt to be acted on, I was once again secured. Let's see, there was a tube down my throat, my mouth was forcibly held open, I had to think to swallow, and my hands were tied down. "Sweet dreams, Mr. Clews."

Whenever my hands were loosened, and I wanted to convey a thought, I tried to write notes. The writing was scrambled and frequently unreadable. I remember a time when my father had an extended ICU stay and had one of those torture tools in his mouth. He was weak and unable to speak. He would try to tell us what he wanted with a scribbled note. We could barely read his once-excellent handwriting. At times, it was so exasperating for him, he would just throw the pencil down and give up. Life's turns are peculiar, aren't they? Here I was decades later, his son, in pretty much the same circumstance.

People would look at my efforts to write, shake their heads, and instinctively ask what I wrote. I would try again. I was thinking desperately, "Please understand what I am trying to say. Please." Dad was gone by then. But you can bet the farm that had he been at that bedside, he would have been the most patient visitor there. Shared experiences breed patience, don't you think? A solution was finally created: I was shown pieces of paper cut out in the form of letters, and I would point to spell out a word. It was usually "water."

It took a couple of days before they removed the torturous device. Of course, that meant pulling out the tube that ran down my throat. Do I need to say I was under for the procedure? I awoke without the tube but with a massive sore throat. My God, the tube must have had scales on it. Every swallow was torturous. And, we all have to swallow. Even those ballplayers who spit all the time still swallow once in a while. I was given medications to try to help soothe the pain. Nothing helped. It does not seem like things are in their natural order when your biggest fear is swallowing. I was offered tepid broth, Jell-O ...

anything that would slide down without scraping. I wanted none of it. If it hurt for slimy saliva to go down, there was nothing on earth that would go down without pain. So I ate nothing. This went on for days. Nothing. *Nada.* One day, a doctor I had not seen before came in. It was around mealtime, and my tray with drinks and easy-to-swallow food was sitting untouched in front of me.

"Why aren't you eating?"

"It hurts to swallow."

"I understand, but you have to eat. Mr. Clews, you're a very weak man, and you need all the nutrition you can get. I want you to eat this lunch."

"I can't. I just don't want it."

"Well, if you don't eat, Mr. Clews, you're going to force us to place a tube up your nose and feed you that way. Do you understand?"

"Could you push that tray closer, please?"

If you think you are tough and nobody will ever tell you what to do, an unpleasant option can do wonders for rethinking how compliant you can be. "We need to do another surgery, or you put this elephant's trunk down your throat." You would be surprised how wide you can open your mouth.

There is not much about life in the ICU that would be described as sociable. There is a certain "go about the business of the day" aura. That is fine when you are so damn beaten that they could bring in candy stripers from "that movie," and your first thought would be, "Do they have to be in here?" But, as I began to swallow without terrible pain and talk without my jaws hurting with every move, I felt my old friendliness coming back. My, as Carol unkindly calls it, "Chatty-Kathy" personality. I may have been Chatty-Kathy but I sounded like Steven Tyler on a bad night.

Of the many differences between ICU and my other hospital homes, one thing particularly bothered me. In my old stomping grounds on Ward 3, for instance, the nurses would linger and chat. But here, not so much. One day, I complained to Carol about what I perceived as the unfriendly nature of the staff.

"There's not a lot of charming bedside manner in here."

"Do you know where you are?"

"Yeah, the ICU."

"And you know what the 'I' stands for, right?"

"Yeah. Insensitive."

Carol disregarded my comeback and, as usual, ignored the punch line. In fact, I did miss the congeniality of the nurses in the CCU. But she was right when she explained how much more moment-to-moment pressure the ICU nurses are under. It was a good day for the nurses if you were not wheeled out with a toe tag.

There was a tech with whom I developed an enjoyable relationship. From my bed, I looked directly at the nurse's station. The particular tech I mention was very friendly. A lot of giving me the Marine, "eyes-focused-on-you" gesture, which always made me laugh. Eventually, I began to do the same to the tech. I felt comfortable being a little more my sometimes bawdy self with this tech. I suspect I made one of those comments during one of Carol's visits. When the tech left the room, Carol chided me for my indiscretion. I told her I always kidded around with him that way.

"Him? Where do you get that?"

"I don't know what you mean."

"Do you think that's a man?"

"Yeah. Sure."

"She's not a man."

"What? Who? No way."

"You haven't been treating her like she's a man, have you? Oh, my God!"

"What makes you think he's a woman?"

"Her name."

Every morning, the nurse and the tech each wrote his or her name on a chalkboard in the room. Carol pointed to the name on the board.

"Read it aloud."

"Carlo."

Carol said nothing but nodded at it again. I looked at it more closely.

"Aw, shit."

I had been misreading it the whole time. I had been seeing the name with an "o" at the end. It was an "a." One stupid letter made all the difference in the world. "How awkward is this?" I realized that I needed to apologize. But this one was going to have to be very carefully phrased. How was I to go about saying to a very nice woman, "I thought you were a man." I gave myself until the next day to think it through. As the gods would have it, she was not on duty the next day. Or the next. And that was the day the transportation folks showed up and I was ushered out of the ICU. I never got to apologize. So now, to that tech: if you are, by some chance, reading this book and recognize yourself in the story, "I'm sorry."

I spent some short time in the PCU and was then shuttled off to the CCU. I was once again back on my old familiar ward. Home, sweet home. I was not put in my old room, but for me the important thing was that I was back with friends. My throat was still pretty painful. I could speak, but my voice continued to be raspy and low. Think Louie Armstrong with a sore throat. I was still on potent antibiotics, and they were making me feel much better. So much in fact that I actually felt like eating. Once I was safely placed in my trusty chair and swallowed some very soft food, it surely felt like hospital home again. The ordeal had taken a toll on me. I was not the only one feeling the results of the marathon. Carol and Ashleigh had been so vigilant about my care that they were running low on energy. Carol came in one day with stains on her clothes. Dark stains. The remnants of a protein chocolate shake she had spilled on herself while driving and drinking her breakfast on the way to work. This was not a happy woman. I think if she could have, she would have grabbed a kitchen knife and performed my transplant right on the spot just to get my hospital stay over and behind us. The best news of the day was that the infection was gone, and I was clear for surgery … if the "exactly right" heart should become available.

Remember the *Saturday Night Live* character Roseanne Roseannadanna and "It just goes to show you. It is always something. If it's not one thing, it is another." The infections, although now gone, had taken a toll on me. I was losing more strength. Even as weak as I was becoming, I was urged to walk. "Stay strong, Mr. Clews." So I decided that as much as I could, I would walk. But weakness was winning the battle, and I did very little to impress my paper slips. I could sense that time was running out. It was now mid-October. July had passed, and then August, September, and now October was slipping by. And still, nothing. Confined to the ward, I began to see myself as a Papillon-like figure. Stuck on this medical island. A scarf around my head. Baggy pants. Dragging a drip stand back and forth to the bathroom. At least Papillon got to have a vegetable garden. Too much time was passing. Here was a "comforting" sentence I heard often: "There are people in here who have been waiting longer than you." There were also people who were not there anymore because they had to wait too long. I tried to find ways to remove thoughts like that from my mind.

I determined early in my diagnosis that I did not want to hear stories from transplant recipients. Every situation was different. I simply did not want to think the transplant was going to be one way only to have it go another and unsettle me. I made the request clear to family, friends, and staff. In spite of that, one day a big woman and her smaller husband on their angel rounds got through to my room. She introduced herself and her survivor mate. She told me that they were there to tell the husband's transplant story. I gently protested and explained my reasoning. I may as well have been talking to my urinal. And so began her *Iliad* of his transplant. The only thing that could have made it more boring was telling it in dactylic hexameter. Well into an hour later, she wrapped it up, and they left. The recipient never said a word. He either understood my request or knew his role. Prop. I do not want to be unfair to the couple. They were nice and thought they were being helpful. After I was fully recovered from my transplant, I offered to be available to the staff, but only if a pending transplant patient wanted to have that conversation. As for the visiting couple, if I had wanted to hear a transplant story, I am sure it would have been helpful. But they should not have made that decision for me.

Do-gooders are different from people who "do good," at least as I see it. People who do good do it where they know they are wanted or needed. Do-gooders cannot be faulted for wanting to help. It just seems that at times, they have no capacity to recognize when their help is not needed or wanted. Or what they are doing.

When I was in Ethiopia, I was told a classic do-gooder's story. I cannot personally vouch for it, but the story was told to me by people who were there when it happened. We were driving from Makele to Axum. I wanted to go to Axum because a group of Coptic monks there claim to have the Ark of the Covenant. I have read enough about the possibilities of its resting place to believe it is there. Visitors to the Church of Our Lady Mary of Zion, where it presumably rests, are not allowed to see the Ark, which was okay with me. I sure as hell did not want to burst into flames. However, we were allowed to stand under it in the basement of the chapel. Do I believe they have it? I do not know for certain, but if they do, I was there. On the way to Axum, we saw six hours of plains, canyons, just a series of absolutely beautiful landscapes. It was dawn as we crossed the plains. I saw farmers' huts with smoke coming through the thatched roofs. The smoke came from burning eucalyptus and smelled wonderful. Of course, smoke filled those huts. I was told that at one point, do-gooders decided that the smoke was unhealthy for the children. So…they worked to have chimneys put in the huts. Suddenly, children began to become ill. It turned out that bugs, once again nesting in the now-smoke-free environment of the thatched roofs, were dropping out and biting children, causing the kiddies to become sick, sometimes fatally so. The chimneys were removed and smoke, once again, filled the roofs. I watched the beauty of things return as they had been, the way the indigenous people knew was best.

Carol missed the guests telling their transplant story I did not want to hear. Given how much time she spent with me, it was a miracle that she was not there for it. I decided to spare her the saga. Outside of a few experiences like that, my stay was beginning to actually have a sense of normalcy. I guess I was beginning to adapt to my circumstances. The nights were still lonely, but I found ways to make them more acceptable. I set some patterns that were not a part of the hospital-suggested ones. For instance, I would wake myself at 2:00 a.m. to watch *Mission Impossible.* I know that sounds crazy but I was going to be awakened around that time anyhow for vitals. Plus, I felt like I was in my very own mission impossible. The days were long and the nights longer. I had to make choices that worked for me to make the best of a bad situation.

Remember the nurse who took us to the races? Before she moved to another hospital, she helped me move to a new room. When she saw the room, she told Carol, "That's the lucky room. The people who go in there wind up getting a heart pretty soon after that."

# Chapter 24
# THE Call

Shortly before midnight on Saturday, October 26, the phone in my room rang. "Mr. Clews, this is Erika Feller. We have a heart for you." Interestingly, I have no idea how I responded.

"Would you like me to call Mrs. Clews, or do you want to?"

"I'll call her."

"Good. The surgery is scheduled for 7:00 a.m. I'll see you before then. Get a good night's sleep."

"Thank you, Dr. Feller. Thank you."

"I'll see you in the morning."

That was it. The call that changed my life. I hung up and dialed our home. Carol picked up and was obviously groggy.

"Vince? Are you all right?"

"Hi, honey. They found a heart."

I heard a scream. And then *click*. And the dial-tone. "What the hell was that?" Just as I started to call Carol back, my cellphone rang. I picked up.

"Did you just call here, or was I dreaming?"

"I called. They have a heart."

"Oh, my God. (through intermittent screaming and sobbing) Thank you, Lord! I'm coming right now. I'll be there as fast as I can. Oh, my God."

"Carol, listen to me. Nothing is going to happen until tomorrow morning. There's no need to rush."

"I'm coming now. Oh, my God. Are you okay? Oh, God. Thank you. Thank you, Lord. I love you, Vince. I'm going to hang up now and get dressed. I love you. Thank you, Lord."

*Click*. Dial tone.

I remember being told that the search for a heart is loosely limited to a 500-mile radius. I guess my rapidly declining condition caused Dr. Feller and her team to extend the normal perimeters. So, on the night of October 26$^{th}$, the team flew to Florida where, sadly, a young man had died. And his family had made the decision to give him new life through others. There must have been some particularly strong indication that we were a cardiac match. According to charts I have seen, the donated heart has four to five hours from cultivation to transplantation. Bear in mind that the team had to run tests when they got to Florida to confirm that the young man and I were the "exactly right" match. If I understand things correctly, that means that while my new heart was in flight, I was being prepped for surgery. The timing for harvesting the heart and preparation for immediate transplant on return required absolute precision. As I was writing this, I was trying to think of an example of that kind of exactitude. In fact, the events surrounding the harvesting and surgery of my transplant *are* the example for the word "exactitude."

On the way to the hospital, Carol starting making calls. Family first. "Italian by injection," as she says. Next, she tried our priest, but he was, sadly, out of town. Then a few friends. And a few enemies. "Na, na, na, na, na, na. He's going to live to keep making your life miserable, you jerk." Okay, the last part is a lie. But I can think of a few people whose night that call would have ruined.

One of the friends Carol called was Dedi. She and Ashleigh got there just about the same time Carol did.

Meanwhile, my room became a beehive of activity. Tests being taken. X-rays. Papers to sign. Of course, we know what they said. In so many words, "By signing here, you agree that if something does go wrong, there will be no lawsuits." I guess if you do not sign those documents, you just lie there and rot. One set of paperwork came with an interesting caution. It read in essence, "Once we have a donor, you are free to decline the heart if there is something about the donor that troubles you."

"'Something about the donor that troubles you?' I am dying here." What in the name of God could there be about a donor that would make me say, "Naw. I'll pass on this one. Let me know when the next one shows up." Any prospective donor would have been screened for a variety of potential problems, like drug use, exposure to AIDS, physical problems that could have damaged the heart, and I do not know what all. Maybe some prospective recipients have been very picky about that sort of thing, but my guess is that they are already dead.

The truth is everything in the documents I was given was explained *ad nauseam*. I felt like I was going to die of boredom before I even got to the OR. While they were talking, my blood was being drawn, and my BP and temperature were being repeatedly taken. In fact, there was so much activity that I gave up following it. I was shaved all the way down and around, if you get my drift. Prep...prep...prep. There was one nice part: beautiful nurses scrubbed down my naked body so I would be hyper-clean for surgery. I was going to ask for the candy stripers to finish the scrub, but it seemed an inappropriate time for that. Everything came to a halt when the surgeons arrived to talk through what was going to happen. They were not too graphic but very thorough.

The anesthesiologist, though, was very specific. I think his paperwork even cautioned about the odds that the induced sleep could become the *big sleep*. I decided not to say anything about my attitude about going under for fear of creeping out the doctor, but I was kind of looking forward to it. I love the feeling of drifting away. That small time when you can feel yourself losing control and it is okay. When I have had to have major dental work done—the kind that you have the option for numbing or for conscious sedation, aka twilight—I take the latter. I would sometimes stop breathing until I would come back to the edge of awareness and breathe deep again so that I could control the sensations. Boy, whenever I did that it would really piss off my oral surgeon. When I was in college, I made the decision not to do drugs. I felt, for various reasons, that I had an addictive personality, so why take the chance? Given my love for twilight, I suspect I was right. If I had started messing around with, say, pot, I probably would have ended up dead, in a gutter somewhere with a needle in my arm.

That did not happen, so I will continue with the burst of activity in my room. I thought about the odds that I would not survive the surgery. All I heard was Ol' Willie singing, "Turn out the lights, the party's over…" I was wrong. The odds were far better that I would come through just fine. No one was turning out the lights. While we were waiting for the transportation team, my nurses and techs, and some of those previously assigned to me, came to visit and wish me well. They hugged Carol. They did not hug me. You know, some things just are not fair. Finally, four-plus months in the hospital surrounded by cute nurses and now with hugs all around, I was too sanitized to be touched. Come on, God.

Carol, Ashleigh, and Dedi all waited with me for the word that it was my turn. We were quiet but not bleak. My new circumstance, even though it involved a complex surgery, was what we had waited for a long time. Interestingly, however, celebration seemed out of place. We chatted for quite some time. Several times, Dedi paused our conversation to pray for me and the doctors and nurses in whose hands my life was being placed. She prayed for peace for my family during the hours to come while they waited for news of the surgery. And, as always, we prayed for the family of the young man whose heart would give me new life. Those were openly emotional moments. Others were just quiet, when no one had much to say. During one of those moments, we suddenly heard a sound that caught everyone's attention: a helicopter was approaching the hospital. Was this the one carrying my new heart? That possibility was cause for momentary speculation. Then back to silence. At one point, I became conscious of the fact that the heart beating in me, the one there since before I was born, was taking some of its last beats in my body. Some of its last beats at all. It would die, and I would live. For those few quiet moments as I thought about that, it felt like I was losing an old and special... very special ...friend.

It was well past 7:00 a.m. when the transportation team showed up to move me to the OR. I got great hugs from Ashleigh and Dedi. I honestly believe none were hugs goodbye. There was a quiet certainty in that room that the next time we saw each other, I would have a new heart, and life would begin anew. My bed was rolled out of the room. As I was being rolled along with Carol following, it occurred to me that should the surgery go bust, the recessional at my funeral might look something like this moment. You know, pallbearers on each side and my family walking behind. Have I said that my funeral is all planned? It will follow the traditional Anglican liturgy. I would be happy if it was an old-fashioned hymn sing with a lot of clapping and foot-stomping to the old revival songs. Pentecostal, early Methodist in fashion. But that is not quite the more traditional service Anglicans prefer. Whatever the rest of the service, I have the ending planned to be as my parents' funerals were. The throng (hey, I can dream) on its feet, the organ playing in honky-tonk fashion the rousing hymn, "When we all get to heaven, what a day of rejoicing that will be." Even if by the time I die I think I am going to hell, I still want the service to end with that hymn. Is that kosher?

The transportation team moved me on what, certainly, was one of the most incredible trips Carol and I had ever taken. Soon we turned a corner, and there were the double doors to *the* room. Carol asked the team if she could have a few moments with me before I was taken in. If I crash through Methuselah's 969 years and live to 1,000, I will never forget what happened next. Carol laid her body across mine and she prayed. She told the Lord she loved me and asked Him to spare me, to bring me back to her. I think there was more, but the sound of the doors opening prohibited me from hearing it. Carol finished her prayer and, knowing the time had come, she leaned up to me, kissed me one more time.

"I love you, Vince."

"I love you, too, honey. I'll see you later."

# Chapter 25
# Joy in the Morning

It was Sunday morning, October 27th. Dedi announced to our congregation that a heart had been found for me and that I was in surgery for the transplant at that very moment. I am told that the entire congregation burst into applause, and prayers of thanks were offered.

Back at the hospital, Carter and Todd joined Carol and Ashleigh. The surgery was scheduled for between four and six hours, give or take. You know how these transplants go. The foursome waited anxiously for any news from the operating room. I was, as always, oblivious to what was going on. If you have not noticed, that is the subtheme of this book. But the OR was hopping. I was asked what kind of music I wanted. I picked Sinatra. How very different this OR was from ones I had seen on my travels. How fortunate we are. I recall in Cambodia seeing a little boy being operated on to release what looked like a giant boil from the middle of his belly. That OR was an open-walled hut. A doctor from the fantastic organization Doctors Without Borders gave him a shot of Novocain and cut. Talk about tough. The little fellow never flinched or cried. Watching it made me feel weak and find a pole to lean on so if I fainted, I would not fall. In my OR, there was music, cleanliness, and comfort. And anesthesia. Blessed anesthesia. It was interesting that there I was, lying on an operating table, ready to have my chest cut open, and once the first shot kicked in, I never gave a second thought to what was going to happen. Amazing.

Because I was not awake for the surgery, trying to describe it in detail would be stupid. So I employed my earlier tactic for information not within my realm of knowledge which, I believe we have seen, is a bit sparse on medical matters. I went to the internet. The University of California San Francisco laid it out at www.ucsf.edu. Forthwith, according to the site's Heart Transplant Procedure page, here is what the surgery involves:

> A major incision down your chest. Your breastbone is split in half.
>
> Your main arteries and veins are connected to a heart lung bypass machine to pump your blood, and a ventilator will help you breathe.
>
> Most heart transplants are done with a method called orthopedic surgery, where most of your heart is removed but the back half of both upper chambers, called atria, are left in place. Then the front half of the donor heart is sewn to the back half of the old heart.
>
> The donor's aorta and pulmonary arteries are connected to yours. The bypass machine is disconnected, and your new heart begins the work of pumping blood.
>
> Your incisions are closed.*

At some point later I was told that before the incision is closed the chest is left open to allow for swelling and to allow access should there be a reason to return to the operating room for additional surgery.

I was an exception for the third item. Note that the back of the heart is left in, and the new heart is attached to that part of the old heart. This is called the *heterotopic technique*. The merging of the two hearts helps the body accept the new organ.

That technique did not work with my heart. It had been too badly damaged by amyloidosis for the back to be used as an anchor. My entire heart had to be removed. One of the surgeons later told Carol that my heart was in the worst condition of any heart he had ever removed...that I should have been dead well before the transplant was even first discussed. Carter may have been Mommy's favorite, but maybe I was God's. So there, Carter.

There is one more item I mentioned earlier worth revisiting. The surgery was scheduled to last four to six hours, the general duration of a heart transplant. I was on the table a little longer. Hey, when you have the stage, play it for all it is worth. That is what I say.

The family waited for news from the operating room in a nice solarium built for angst. No news was expected for at least four hours. Because it was major cardiac surgery, there was good reason to be tense. The attending family kept busy keeping other family members up-to-date. The clock seemed to move slowly, like it was playing games with the situation. When the fourth hour passed, then hour five and no word from the OR, some anxiety began to set in.

Even with the great trust the staff at UMMC justifiably had earned with the Clews family, by hour six, things had gone from tense to stressed. Seven. Ashleigh called her nurse friend, Cosene, who worked with the Cardiac Unit, to see if she could find out what was going on. She did. And she reported back that there was some trouble with heavy bleeding. Eight. Nine hours. No word. None. Ten. Ten hours and nothing. Late in the eleventh hour, the doctors came out to talk to my waiting family. Everyone there later said the surgeons looked like they had been hit by a truck. The first question: "Is he okay?"

"Yes."

The transplant was finished, and all signs were that it was successful. The new heart was in, and my body was accepting it. The doctors confirmed what the family had heard. Excessive bleeding created problems that caused the surgery to last longer than usual. They were told that several times, I came close to bleeding out. It is always something, isn't it? Excessive bleeding. I have never been good with the sight of blood. I am surprised I did not faint right there on the table. Before the doctors left, they arranged for my family to visit me in the ICU. Carol and Ashleigh were the first to come to see me. Each took a hand, and as I had when I recognized their presence after the most recent sepsis incident, I squeezed their hands. "I'm here. I made it." Carol noticed that my hands were warm for the first time in several years. New heart, warm hands.

Weeks earlier, in anticipation of a successful transplant, Carter had made a purchase for the event:

T-shirts. He had ordered them from Duck Dynasty just for this moment. The T-shirts read:

>Happy
>Happy
>Happy

*I obtained the surgeon's oral report on the transplant surgery. For those who care to read it, and are smart enough to understand it, I have included a reformatted version in the Appendix.

# Chapter 26
# Alive and Aware…
# Well, Alive

Everyone was happy. Maybe even me. Of course, if I was, I did not know it. If, by some freak of nature I had known, I am sure I would have wanted a "Happy" T-shirt, too. The problem then would have been that it would have not fit properly over my open chest. And we know how I am about the way my clothes look on me.

Here I was. A newborn at seventy years old. How about that? For once in my life I was actually an answer to prayer. I had become the successful beneficiary of a heart transplant. All the prayers and good wishes that a heart would be found in time, and those for a successful surgery, had been answered. Now the advocates were praying a prayer of a different kind. Actually, it was more like a jukebox of thanks for a successful surgery. Of thanks for a special medical team who cared for me from the beginning of my cardiac crisis right through the surgery. And there were prayers for a full recovery. Prayers for strength for Carol, Ashleigh, and the rest of the family. And, of course, prayers of thanks for the donor family who expressed their love for one of their own in such a selfless way. Through grief, joy. What a remarkable gift.

When the doctors felt comfortable that it was time to shuttle me off to others for care, I was moved to the ICU. I have written about the intensive care I have received when I was moved there on other occasions. I cannot imagine the attention on this visit being any more concentrated than during my prior stays. Of course, on those occasions they were keeping me from dying. Now the team was keeping me alive. I know that sounds like six of one and half a dozen of another. But, for patients in that room, the former is, "I'm slipping. Don't let me fall." The latter is, "I'm climbing. Help pull me up."

As I drifted in and out of my induced slumber, I found out that the doctors had added insult to injury. Not only had they opened my chest, they also had opened my mouth…and stuck a ventilator in it. "For God's sake, spare me that insult." Happily, the experience was short-lived. I had no clue what else was going on, but I was lucid enough to start breathing through my nose. I was able to pass the test for removal of the squatter. The mouth monster was removed within the day. That was followed by the obligatory painful throat. In short order, the pain was aggravated further by insistence that I cough to keep mucus from going into my lungs. Cough? Cough? My chest had just been split open. It hurt to think.

I am not saying I was special and, I suspect, we know it is standard operating procedure in ICU, but I was given the kind of singular attention folks at the Ritz wish they would get. On each shift, I had my own nurse, one assigned especially to me. Aside from that, I suppose I was treated like any other heart-transplant patient. I was monitored 24/7. My blood pressure, oxygen level, breathing rate, and heart rate were all on the radar. Blood samples were taken regularly to monitor the status of the new heart, my lungs, liver and, of course, those rascally kidneys. There were X-rays to make sure my heart was beating to the beat. I was on IVs dripping medications, which the nurses were also monitoring. The men who walked on the moon were probably monitored less. Of course there was constant attention to make sure I was not having any reactions to the drugs. And I was on plenty. I was on anti-rejection meds to help fight my body's natural inclination to reject the new organ. "Come on, guys. We need a little 'welcome mat' thing going on here, please." The whole time they were doing all this, they were watching for any sign of an infection. This was not a good time for a reappearance of sepsis. I am telling you, they watched over me like I was royalty. When will that happen again in my life? Here is the kicker. I was completely out of it and missed the whole damn thing. May I say, as the guy who was cut open, whose sternum was broken just a day before this and now sleeping comfortably a night later, those drugs should never be available on the streets.

When Carol and Ashleigh were convinced that I was out of any danger, they left. It was now time for them to spend some time recovering after all the months of adjusting lives to be my daily support. They were justifiably exhausted. When Carol arrived home, and before she could even put her purse down, Simon came from where he was lying by my chair and wanted to know how I was doing and all the details of the day. That dog. Simon, for all our rides in the Thing, was Carol's dog. I am certain that before she did much else, she gave him some well-deserved attention.

Actually, none of what you just read after "justifiably exhausted" is true, except that Simon was Carol's dog. I wish what I wrote was true. Here is what really happened that night: Carol arrived home to an empty house. You see, shortly after I was admitted to the hospital with my life hanging in the balance, Simon's age began to catch up with him. Todd had decided that he should stop by the house on long days and make sure Simon was fed, had water, and got some exercise. He spent time giving the good old dog some of the human attention he had been used to. One evening when Carol arrived home, he broke the news to her that poor old Simon's physical and mental capabilities were just about exhausted. Carol was heartbroken but agreed with Todd that it was time. They arranged for a mobile pet-care unit to come to the house. Carol sat on the floor and held her Simon as his pain was gently relieved, forever. From that day until I was released from the hospital months later, Carol came home each night to an empty house. A dark, empty house. There was then, and still is, a magnet on the refrigerator that reads, "God gives us no more than we can handle." I suspect there were nights when it took all of Carol's spiritual strength not to grab that magnet and throw it right into the trash.

Carol was there every day until she finally had to go back to work. I hated the thought that she was not going to be with me. However, the time had come for her to begin to normalize her life. The same for Ashleigh. Once the main crisis was over, Carol returned to the pattern of work, hospital, home, and so on. There was a difference this time, though. Her life no longer revolved around a phone call from the hospital with one of two messages: "Mrs. Clews, I'm sorry to inform you…" or "We've found a heart." Sometime after I had fully recovered, she told me about a day when she was driving to work and began to yell. Just yell. Then that turned into a scream, which became one unbridled scream after another. It was such an unrestrained release that she had to pull over, put the car in park, and let herself scream and scream until it was out of her. She had had it. When I related this event to my remarkably well-read brother, Carter cited a passage from Richard Nixon's book *Six Crises*. Like Nixon or not, the man knew about crises: "The toughest time in a crisis is after the danger passes. It is then that the adrenaline has stopped flowing, the fatigue sets in, and you finally give out."

I spent ten days in ICU. Carol, of course, was there every day. What a lousy way to eat up your sick leave and vacation days. The attention I received from the doctors and ever-present nurses mended me well enough to move on to my next stop on the way home. They did everything they could but stop the pain.

When I was well enough, I was moved to a step-down unit. Pretty simply, a step-down unit is an area of the ICU where the patient requires less scrutiny (i.e., less attention to Vince). Because I felt insecure and weak, I raised an objection to leaving ICU. Nonetheless, I was to be moved. Dumb me to resist. In stepping down, I also stepped closer to home.

One factor that helped Carol survive the intensity and crises was the outstanding support from the staff around her at work. The folks redoubled their efforts to give her the time she required to be the support I needed. Staff, board members, and volunteers redoubled their effort. And, of course, they all prayed. On one occasion, while I was still in ICU, I awoke long enough to see a priest sitting in a chair near my bed. He smiled, and I fell right back to sleep. When I next awoke, he was still there. I have no idea how long he just sat at my bedside. Fr. Joe was the priest at one of the many Roman Catholic churches that supported Carol's organization. He is a loving, and very funny, friend who had come to pray and bring encouragement. Still, in my situation, lying in an all-white room, with my vision blurred, and a priest praying at my bedside, I just assumed that maybe things had gone wrong. My clue to reality was that in my awake moments, I was in pain.

Carol and Ashleigh got an extended reprieve from their daily visits when Marcia and Ernie, my sister and her husband, spent several days with me. They would come in mid-morning and stay until sometime after dinner. I cannot recall why, but at that time, I fell into an exaggerated melancholy mood, the kind that makes you feel like you are perpetually caught on the verge of tears. Maybe it was having my little sister there. For instance, when they would leave each night, I felt a loneliness I cannot describe. It was the same type of heaviness I often felt when Carol would leave. There is actually something called *post-cardiac surgery depression*. Whatever it was, it was so bad that it hovered like low fog most of the night. I experienced that same feeling on one of Carter's visits. It was a feeling of loneliness and despair unusual to my stay. I asked him to spend the night. I could see that he really did not want to do it. But he did. Because there was only one bed, he spent the night in the room's recliner. I happily would have slept there, but I was prisoner to the bed. The next morning, he explained that he loved me but that he had spent his last overnight at the hospital. "I'm never doing that again. Between the nurses coming in and out all night and the lousy chair, that's the worst night of sleep I've ever gotten."

The chair was exactly like the one I had spent days, and many nights, sleeping in during my pre-surgery months. I loved sleeping in it. Maybe I had gotten used to the peculiar curvatures from months and months of slumbering, first in the one at home, and then later in the hospital version. As for the nurses' comings and goings, I was so conditioned to the patterns that I could sleep right through them. Unless they wakened me for a particular purpose, I often slept right through their visits. Carter was good to his word. He visited often but never again spent the night.

When I began to get stronger I also began to get hungry. How about that? So bring on some eggs over easy, pan-fried potatoes, and scrapple. No toast. I am watching my weight. No need to worry about that, as it turned out. Once again, I could barely swallow my own spit. And I was not going to be allowed to eat until they were sure I could comfortably swallow. I guess the idea of another trip to the OR to cut my throat open just to retrieve an errant piece of pan-fried potato was not part of cardiac surgery recovery. A nurse, whom I suppose specialized in swallowing, tested my capability and, nope, not there yet. When I was five years old, my tonsils were removed. I remembered being allowed to have ice cream while I sat on a stool in my Aunt Molly's kitchen. I watched the corner stoplight change and ate ice cream. Her version of post-op was a lot more fun than the one after the transplant.

When it was determined that I was strong enough, and, I guess, would not fall open all over the bed, I was returned to the CCU. I returned to a room looking much like the one I left to go to the OR for my heart transplant. In fact, it may have been the same one. I might have known for sure except the buildup of anesthesia from the surgery and the drugs had me pretty much in a fog. Thank God.

I have read that we do not remember what pain feels like. There are times, though, that I think we do. Maybe much more right after the incident that caused it. I have, at times, in this book described how I thought the pain felt. But, it is all from some memory of the incident. But my mind never let me re-create the feeling of the pain in a way that I could feel it again. Good fortune for a writer writing about painful experiences. A blessing for all of us.

Whether it was post-surgical cognizance or mind-bending drugs, or both, I was definitely struggling when one day several weeks after I was comfortably back in the CCU, I decided to call Carol. I picked up the phone, but I could not remember her office phone number. Not at all. Not her cell, nor our home number.

I did not know where we lived. In fact, I could not remember exactly what was going on outside my room. I knew I was in the hospital, but I was confused about life outside it. I did not know my home address. I did not know squat. The fog went on for the whole day. When Carol came in, I told her that earlier I wanted to call her but could not recall any of her phone numbers. "In fact," I told her, "I can't remember our other phone numbers or where we live or much about the outside world." Carol got some paper and a pen and wrote all the critical information on it. As she wrote some of it, I recognized the information. But too much of it was still unclear for Carol's liking. She spoke to several of the nurses.

"Have you noticed instances where Vince seems out of it?"

"Probably the same thing you've seen, Mrs. Clews. He's still going to have some holdover effects from the anesthesia. He was under for a long time."

"I've read something about that. As I recall it said that he could be affected for about two weeks for every hour he was under."

"Around that."

"And you add the pretty heavy stuff he's taking now."

"Oxycodone."

"Maybe he's asking for too much of it. Maybe that's a problem."

"Well, he asks for it pretty regularly. But don't worry. He's allotted only so much. But his circumstances could be a contributor to his fogginess."

That evening, after Carol left, I noticed a familiar handwriting on the whiteboard where the nurses and techs left messages for each other. It read, "No more oxycodone for Vince." I studied the note on the board. Yes. Yes. The handwriting was Carol's. I pushed my call button.

"Could I see a nurse or a tech, please?"

A nurse came in.

"Do you see that note on the board about the drugs?"

"The note about the oxycodone?"

"Yes, that one."

"Carol wrote that. I recognize her handwriting. You can just erase it."

The nurse, who knew us from earlier times with us, laughed.

"Erase it?"

"Yes. I love her and hope she never has any experience with pain even remotely like I'm having. But if, God forbid, that ever happens, then she can have you write that on her whiteboard. Right now it's my pain and my board, so you can just erase it."

At that moment, I did not see Carol as much of a patient advocate and surely not "the good wife." At that moment, not a caring wife. For only that moment.

Neither my thoughts, nor Carol's for that matter, had any bearing on my drug allotments. It was all prescribed. The issue was dropped. As the pain became less severe, I needed less help to tolerate it. There were moments, though, when I wished I was still feeling nothing. Some of the tasks that needed to be done around me were reminders that I had undergone surgery, and the pain still could be really bad. For instance, when they changed the sheets, there was no escaping knowing they were doing it. And, like some kind of clean freaks, they did it every day. They tried to be careful, but they had to roll me from side to side to get the old sheets off and then the clean ones on the bed. Oh, my God, did it hurt. The roll was painful enough. Once they got me in position lying on one side, the weight of the upper side of my body laid directly on my sternum. And the sternum was trying to hold its own against totally collapsing from the weight bearing down on it. I have always heard that bones do not have nerves, but there was no way, during those painful minutes, you could have convinced me that was true. Something hurt like nobody's business right where my incision was. And it was my nerveless sternum. The bedding change lasted three, maybe four minutes…or hours.

On those occasions when I had messed the bed, and sadly my initial immobility made that happen too often, the procedure took even longer. It hurt so much. And I do believe that the humiliation of a mortifying experience adds to the pain.

Because things were going smoothly, it was time for another bout with real pain, only this time where I least expected it. It began with a wheelchair ride to get an X-ray. Let me tell you, I was X-rayed so much during my stay that I set off Geiger counters at an archeology dig ten miles away. The process of getting me out of bed into a wheelchair could be summed up in a single phrase: "Just shoot me."

On one occasion transportation took me somewhere a long way from my room for an X-ray.

It was taken, and I was left in the hall for pickup. I waited and waited and then waited some more. The X-ray folks finished their shift and closed down. I asked them to call Transportation. They either did and it was disregarded, or they did not call. I waited some more. In a short time, it seemed the area of the building where I was was vacated—and cold. I was in my bathrobe, but I was getting colder and colder. And very lonely. I began to wonder if anyone was going to figure out that I was missing. I would have wheeled myself back to my room, but I had no idea where I was. Let's face it, one could get lost for a pretty long time in a building big enough to have rooms for 3,000 people. It was not long before my chest and back both were beginning to hurt from sitting upright for so long. I would shift to help ameliorate the pain, but that did not help much. Trust me, those wheelchairs are not designed for patient comfort. Meanwhile, back at my empty room, Carol came for a visit. She set the alarm.

"Where's Vince?"

Somewhere in limbo, I continued my hiatus as the man without a ride. The most I could do to make myself comfortable was to make a slight shift in position. As time went on, shifting became more difficult and painful. I injured my back when I was in high school, and several times subsequent to that and it's not my friend. Sit still and in a short time it hurts. Move, and it hurts to move. "Where is some one? Just one anyone." Pain and isolation created an increased sense of despair. I do not know how long I sat in that chair. After quite some time a Transportation person showed up. The excuse:

"We're really busy." Thank God surgery was not run like transportation.

"Doctor, the patient is sedated, chest open and waiting on the operating table."

"Just leave him there. I'm busy. I'll be around later."

My chair was unlocked, and we began the journey home. At some point along the matrix of halls and elevators, Carol and Sean, who had begun a trek to the X-ray area where I had been wasting away, found me. When I got back to the room and started to get out of the wheelchair, I felt serious pain in my lower back. Of course, that was bound to happen. The amount of time I spent immobilized in a wheelchair would make Superman's back hurt. Getting from the chair to my bed was slow and excruciating. After some adjusting—painful adjusting—I was in my bed and on my back. Now all I had to do was stay right there in that position for a few days until they would send me home. I knew one thing for certain: I was never again going to let myself be carted from my room without my cellphone and a set of phone numbers to call for help. I never needed to use them. It was one bad incident among scores and scores of good ones during my stay at UMMC.

As the surgery event, and the errant wheelchair time, were further behind me, I became more comfortable. I asked for fewer pain medications. One day, I asked that they give me no painkillers at all. I wanted to be alert and as close to being my old self as possible. You see, Carol had notified me that she had, once again, arranged to spend the night. Of course, being Ms. Modesty, she had ordered a second bed. I told the staff to act like they never heard her. Sadly, she had established herself as the voice of reason. Even authority. So, I went straight to Carol with my case.

"Why do we have to have a second bed? We can share a single. I'm well now."

"I know. That's why I'm getting my own bed. I don't trust you one bit."

"I'm not that healthy yet. I can't do anything."

"No way. You are your grandfather's grandson."

"What the hell's that supposed to mean?'"

I knew what it meant. My grandmother Marciano complained to my mother that Grandad, then well into his eighties, kept bothering her about sex. He wanted to do it. Mom told her, "Don't worry. He can't do anything." To which Grandmother replied, "Like hell he can't." I got most of my traits from the Clews side of the family. That night, I prayed like a tent preacher for one night of Marciano blood to surge into first place.

Carol changed in the bathroom, got into my bed for a short time, and went back to her bed for the night. Hell, we may as well have been home with me in the downstairs chair. What was the point of getting a new heart? I knew the answer to that question. Because there was *"a time a comin'"* when she will be getting undressed and I will be home, and the downstairs chair finally will be empty.

# Chapter 27
# Back on My Feet?

Dr. Christiaan Barnard wrote, "Suffering isn't ennobling, recovering is ennobling." I agree.

By all measures, my recovery was going fine. Heart beating strong. Kidneys bouncing back. Swallowing real food. Fog clearing. Thumb less attached to the call button.

It was now early November, and our thoughts were turning to Thanksgiving. Mine were turning in a big, exciting way. It is my favorite holiday. Thanksgiving. Rare is the person in this country who does not have something to be thankful for. I sure did. All indications were that I would be at my place at head of the table, alive and well. The Patriarch. The most elder. Head of the family. I like that distinction. Although I would gladly have passed it back to Dad.

Thanksgiving. It had been a rough year, but, I was going to be home for the big day. I was sure of that. And thankful. Real thankful. Actually, it should not have taken lifesaving surgery to make me feel thankful. I had seen enough hunger and suffering to make me more than grateful for what I have. I have been at food-distribution centers where people waited hours for just a bag of grain. I remember visiting a refugee camp in Angola where people lived in filth, and expectations of food were day to day. I saw hungry children. I saw what hunger does to their little bodies. As I look at celebrities who have made rail-thin a standard for beauty, I wonder if they have ever seen that look when there is nothing chic about it. The blindness to the reality of the "look" is incomprehensible. It is not chic. It is sick.

I seem for some reason, at times, to have turned this book into a platform. No apology. But I will get back to the story.

It is interesting how you can overlook the obvious. If I was going to go home, I was going to have to be able to walk. My assumption had been all along that I would be going back to Kernan for a short rehabilitation, specifically to teach me to walk again on my now very-much-weakened legs. As anxious as I was to go home, I wanted to walk into the house, not arrive in a wheelchair. Kernan. That was the plan. As President Dwight Eisenhower wrote, "Plans are nothing."

One morning two men walked in and announced they were there to help me walk. "I don't think so." I had barely moved out of bed at that point. And even then, and with extensive help, only to step from the bed onto a scale to be weighed. They did that every day. A nurse and tech helped me out of bed directly onto the big, roll-in scale. They would hold me up while the scale was set to weigh me. Then they would have to let go and balance me while the scale did its obscene duty. I would try to stay standing, which I could do only for a few seconds or so until they had the weight, and then I slumped into my bed, which was directly behind me. It was a painful and demoralizing experience. Well, not all demoralizing.

My weight was in the low 180s. "The low 180s." I did not even know weight that low existed in my world anymore. I could not wait to get home to my clothes. I was not going to have to unbutton my pants after my Thanksgiving pumpkin pie.

The two men who had entered my room turned out to be physical therapists.

"Mr. Clews, right?"

I knew about physical therapy and wanted none of it. Even though I knew the outcome was worth it, the idea of starting it again and going through the pain was not something I was prepared for.

"No. I believe you're supposed to be in another room. I think he's two doors down. A much younger man. Off you go."

Nope. They were not buying it. They had with them what looked like a walker, but it was taller. After a few niceties, they turned back to business.

"Okay, Mr. Clews, we're going to get you out of that bed, and you're going to do some walking."

My further protest went without regard. They put on my slippers. Then they moved the walker to the bed. In mid-protest, I was hoisted to my feet.

"I can't stand. My legs... wait, wait."

"There you go. Now, put your arms on the walker. Put them up there and lean on them."

The therapists put my arms on the walker. As soon as they were raised and my weight rested on the walker, I felt a sharp pain in my chest. My arms slid right off. I slumped right back into the bed. I had no legs. Well, I had legs. I had seen "no legs." I had legs. They just were not working.

The gentlemen were going to help me use my fragile legs, whether I was ready or not. They assisted me back up onto the walker. I was leaning on my arms with little help from my legs. My arms had had almost as little exercise as my legs. That is, unless we count lifting a cup of pudding three times a day. The men surrounded me and began to help me move. Wait, who was I kidding? They moved me. I was being moved away from the bed and forward, insisting the whole time that I help. I doubt very much that my legs were at all involved, but we moved to the door. Listen, the last thing I want to portray myself as is a crybaby. But for some reason, I recall crying out that I could not do what they wanted. It was not so much that my legs would not move. My chest felt like it was going to split like a dried piece of wood. It hurt, and that was scaring the daylights out of me. I had visions of a sudden crack, a tearing sound, my gown turning bloody, and my heart plopping out onto the floor. They moved me back to the bed. I sat there for a moment completely rattled. The nurse took my vitals. She was damn lucky there were any to take. The men waited and then turned toward the door.

"You relax. You did fine. We'll see you later today." And they meant it. Waiting for them was a harrowing experience. But not as harrowing as going through the same thing I had earlier. This time, the weight was on my legs…and feet. As my feet began to feel the weight, pain shot through them. The bottoms of my feet felt like I was standing on knives, sharp edge up. A lot of knives cutting through pins and needles. I had been feeling numbness in my feet since I began to feel again. It was an extreme numbness that, contrary to the description, created a peculiar form of discomfort even while they were at rest. It turned out it was due to neuropathy. The following description from Answers.com is pretty close to what I was experiencing on the bottoms of my feet: "Neuropathic pain is usually perceived as a steady burning and/or 'pins and needles' and/or 'electric shock' sensations. The difference is due to the fact that 'ordinary' pain stimulates only pain nerves, while a neuropathy often results in the firing of both pain and non-pain (touch, warm, cool) sensory nerves in the same area, producing signals that the spinal cord and brain do not normally expect to receive." "Welcome to being back on your feet, Mr. Clews. We've been waiting for you."

This pain was complicated by another issue that had developed with my feet while I was bedridden. There is a kind of crusty coating, like one deep foot-shaped callous on the sole of each foot that keeps the nerve endings from directly touching, say, the floor. My crusty soles had gone AWOL and were not going to return. So what was touching the floor with each step was, basically, nerve endings. That hurt (and still does) with almost every step. Sometimes it even hurt when my feet were not touching anything. Here is an irony: my heart is now strong enough to walk for exercise. My feet hurt enough for me not to do it.

If that day of trying to walk was any indication of what was to come, the nurse who had earlier lectured me on post-transplant pain hit it right on the head: "You don't know what real pain is. You just wait until you've had a transplant. Then you'll find out what pain is."

Guess what? She may have been mean and verbally ugly, but she was right.

# Chapter 28
# Christmas, Too?

There are several actors whose work I particularly enjoy. Bill Murray is high on the list. Of course, it does not hurt that he did a film titled *St. Vincent*. He also was in a film with a piece of dialogue that perfectly described my attempt to walk: "Baby steps," from the very funny movie *What About Bob?*

You know what baby steps will not get you? Home for Thanksgiving. Carol saw the issue approaching and decided to bring Thanksgiving dinner to the hospital. She booked a conference room on the ward. Her plan was to bring the dinner, the family, and all the festivities to me, and to include anyone on Ward 3 that could stop in. However, it became apparent that the complications involved to use the room for the feast were overwhelming. She was distressed by the idea that I would spend my favorite holiday alone, in a hospital to boot. So was I. The hospital was going to serve turkey with the usual trimmings. But it was more than the meal that I loved about Thanksgiving. For instance, I was going to miss watching Carol fixing the dinner.

I knew Carol long before we were married. I always had this fantasy about her. Yeah, that one, too. But I saw her as Beaver Cleaver's mother. You know, June Cleaver in *Leave It to Beaver*. June Cleaver. If you have never bathed in the comfort of watching 1950s and early-'60s TV family sitcoms,

CHRISTMAS, TOO?

do yourself a favor. Wander Mayberry. Have dinner with the Cleavers. Visit a member of the Andersons' home. Of course, there were things about that decade that diminish the glow. But as a child of the '50s, I can affirm that there was "a kinder, gentler society."

As I said, I used to fantasize that Carol prepared Thanksgiving dinner dressed like Mrs. Cleaver. Heels, a close-fitting skirt, cashmere sweater, pearl necklace, and a nice apron. Preparing Thanksgiving dinner dressed just as she would spend the rest of the day. Yeah, I know. Well, it was not quite like that. Just being home with her would have been better than any fantasy. But it was not to be so this year. On top of that, I was not going to get to experience the joy I always felt being with my family on that very special day. On Thanksgiving Day that year, members of the family visited my room throughout the morning. Their visits maintained the sense of family I was otherwise going to miss. Because the hospital was going to serve turkey and the trimmings, I asked Carol if she instead would bring me some crab cakes, which she did. Crab cakes and the trimmings. Happy Thanksgiving.

Shortly after Thanksgiving I was thinking about Christmas. So was anyone who watched TV. Shoot, we had been thinking about it since before Halloween when the merchandisers started running 1-800 TV ads for gift return centers.

I love Christmas carols. I like them so much that every year in July, I slip some Christmas CDs into my car CD player. In the middle of the heat and humidity, I put the top down on my convertible and drive down the road listening to "White Christmas" or any one of the myriad Christmas songs I just love. You know what happens when you pull your car into a shopping-center parking lot with the top down and "Jingle Bells" blaring from your radio in the heat of summer? You can pick your parking space. People think you are nuts and move to a spot down the lot. I love Christmas music more than any other music. I have a long-standing tradition that from the day after Thanksgiving, I play only Christmas music until January 2nd. Radio, CDs, Pandora—whatever the source, it is the music of the season. Carol loves the songs and carols but loses her enthusiasm for the round-the-clock version. You have to wonder how couples with a difference of that sort stay together, don't you?

At some point during my recovery, Carol gave me a radio. I kept the radio in the bathroom playing a classical music station, 24/7. That changed the day after Thanksgiving. In Baltimore, there is one radio station that, post-Thanksgiving, plays nothing but the music of the magical Christmas season until the beginning of the New Year. God bless the owners' hearts. All who entered my room heard carols and songs that made you want to open gifts. I later found out that my little radio was the only one on the ward playing seasonal music. The nurses moved the portable computer table next to the door to my room so they could hear the seasonal songs and carols while they worked. The music also indicated that it was getting colder outside which, interestingly enough, made me colder inside. It was just about this time that my then-daughter-in-law, Mara, presented me with a beautiful blanket. Blue and white. I loved it. It was so comfortable that I never used a hospital blanket the rest of my stay.

At some point between holidays, I realized that even if I was released from the hospital before Christmas, I was not going to be able to go shopping. I am not one of those people who loves to shop and wrap. They are usually the ones who are so organized that, by November 1st, they are finished. I have always liked the experience of buying presents that I knew were going to make the recipient happy. I enjoyed going past department-store windows that were decorated with Christmas themes, sometimes with moving mannequins. I loved the smell of the big stores and riding the escalator. Well, I still do. But none of that was going to matter if I was still in the hospital.

I called Ashleigh.

"Will you help me do some of my Christmas shopping?"

"Sure. Give me a list."

"I think I can buy some of it from stuff I see on TV."

"Don't do that. You'll screw it up. Just give me a list."

She was right. I would have screwed it up. We decided at one point that the extended family was so big that buying gifts for everyone was breaking our piggybanks. So among the adults, we drew names. Of course, I still wanted to get Carol several gifts. Ashleigh volunteered to do my shopping. A big question for me was this: how to get Carol the sexy piece or so of clothing I always liked to get her...for me to see her in when I got home. Asking Ashleigh to shop for that just did not sound cricket. I gave Ashleigh a list, absent anything that would embarrass her, which she obligingly bought and wrapped. Of course, there was this: Where were we going to be when I gave Carol and my Secret Santa their gifts? I did not want Christmas to be another Thanksgiving. Spending holidays in a hospital sucks.

# Chapter 29
# "If You Can Wait and Not Be Tired by Waiting"*

My hospital stay had now worked its way well into December. We were nearly six months into it by then. That would be all of July, all of August, all of September, all of October, all of November, and now it was December. I write "we" because my family was going through it with me, as witnessed by the utter disruption in Carol's life and all the adjustments Ashleigh had to make in hers. There were Carter's four-hour round-trip visits. Marcia and Ernie and Keith and Ingrid had come back and forth from Kentucky and Tennessee. Donna and Jay had driven from Wisconsin. Friends like Mike had visited almost every day. And others such as Griff, Dedi, Patrick, Charlie, and Dick were so regular the nurses knew them on sight.

For years before my hospitalization, Griff, Ralph, and AJ were adjusting schedules to get me to doctors' appointments. It had gone on too long, and now here I was, still stuck in the hospital. The question was, was it going to be all of December? It was hard to believe that I ever read, "After the surgery, you typically will spend one to two days in the recovery room, two to three days in the intensive care unit, and about seven days in the transplant unit." That is from cedar-sinai.org. It is pretty much in line with everything else I read. Can you understand that the extended stay, accompanied by no declared end, was all beginning to get frustrating?

Timely. That is what some things were. One day, Carol brought in a small shipping box with some get-well cards. I opened it and, among the cards, there was a framed picture sent by Allen Scheid, a client, and friend, with whom I had traveled to some of the destinations I mention in this book. The picture was of a handmade wooden fishing boat, sitting in the foreground with other similar boats along a shoreline. The boat had a worn message painted across it—one word: Perseverance. I mentioned earlier that I had traveled to a number of countries. The assignments were for two organizations that, like so many NGOs, do wonderful work. Most of the countries we visited were what were then called "developing nations." One of them was Sierra Leone in Africa. Sierra Leone is beautiful. On the Atlantic. White sand beaches. Green mountains that touch the shoreline. We were told that there was no airport on the mainland, so our plane landed on an island several miles from the shoreline. We were given two choices to get to the mainland. The first was by ferry. Our host told us that the ferries had a bad reputation for sinking. The ferry was out. The alternative was to fly on one of two very old Russian troop helicopters. There were no seats. We sat along the side of the chopper on metal "benches." We lifted off. The thing shook so badly that I was absolutely confident we were going to drop right into the water. There were three nuns sitting across from me. They were saying the Rosary frantically, it seemed to me, the whole flight. I am not Catholic, but I crossed myself right along with them when our ride landed safely on the continent.

One of our stops on the mainland was a fishing village made up of small huts. The tiny community sat at the ocean's edge. It was so very peaceful. It appeared that there was nothing there to invite the clatter and chaos of the outside world. It was idyllic. A place we dream about. An unrefined Shangri-La. There was one reminder, however, that daily life is the same everywhere. Even where it looks like an escape, it isn't. Perseverance. I kept the photo Allen sent me where I could see it for the rest of the stay as a reminder of my role in my recovery.

A lengthy hospital stay, it turns out, can make a person do things he or she has never done before. For me, it was buying things I saw on infomercials. One day, Carol sprung a surprise question: "Where's the credit card?"

"What credit card?"

"Come on. Hand it over. The one you've been using to buy all that crap that keeps arriving at the house."

You know, it is amazing how those TV guys can make it seem like you absolutely have to have that six-hotdogs-at-a-time cooker. Maybe we did not need that. But it made sense to me that Carol should have the LED lanterns for the house if power was lost while I was in the hospital. Some of the other things I cannot justify. The stuff never worked. What was funny was that I used to produce TV infomercials, so I had some idea that you often do not get what you think you bought. Well, maybe you do. It just does not work the way they told you it would.

Toward the end of my stay there was an incident, though begun with good intentions, that did not work out as well as was intended. It was a haircut. By the time I had been in that hospital for all those months, I looked like a mad prophet who had been wandering the wilderness for years. Long, unruly, now gray hair. Scraggly gray beard. Carol decided to fix that. On the recommendation of a friend, she hired a young woman "stylist" to cut my hair. That sounded good. She showed up one day while Carter was visiting and began her attack. She was talking about how good she was while she chopped away. I like a full head of hair and really did not mind that it was considerably unruly from the long hospital stay. Getting it cut was a courtesy to Carol. As Carter watched the "stylist" chatting away while she chopped at my hair, he held up a picture of Carol and me.

"Uh, this is how my brother wears his hair. Full and curly."

The slasher babbled on about a previous hair-butchering she had done.

"Even while I was cutting his hair, he was saying it was the best haircut he had ever been given."

I knew of the fellow she was babbling about. He wore a buzz cut. Carter tried again.

"You can see that he likes it full and a little long. See, right here in the picture.

"He said he was prouder of the haircut than all those awards he's ever won."

I knew something was terribly wrong when Carter put the picture down and shook his head. My formerly full, bushy hair was now short and straight. It was such a bad haircut that even the nurses could not stop themselves from commenting. You talk about, once again, adding insult to injury.

On the good-news side, the walking instructors had done their job well. In almost no time, I had retrieved my old friends—the "paper walking slips"—and was touring the circumference of the ward. At first, it was a matter of moving from the tall walker to my regular one. I had some of the same kind of fears then that I had about moving from the bed to the big walker. What if my arms gave out? My legs certainly were not strong enough to keep me upright by themselves. Just as it had been with every "first time" move on the earlier recovery road, attempting to walk was challenging. I was actually taking some steps. I began to spend a part of my days in a nearby rehab room working on real steps. Up and down them. Six of them. That accomplished, I spent time out in the hall, trying the hospital steps, with the help of my therapist. Yep. No problem. In no time up twelve, holding onto the railing for dear life, of course. Soon I was walking on my own. Climbing stairs. Dancing. Well, maybe not that. But I was feeling good and comfortably mobile. The stay was almost over. I was ready to get back to normalcy.

Then again, maybe not. My post-surgery fluid buildup was not dropping the way it should have. I thought this type of thing was in the past. But no. Here it was, another fluid issue. It was just as if I never went through years of discomfort, setbacks, challenges, and medical procedures to address the problem. No pain. No perceived recovery. It was as if I never spent five months in the hospital. No transplant. No ICU. Nothing. It now seemed that no amount of diuretics could curb the buildup. Control it, yes. But only to a degree.

If you think I was being a little obsessive, try spending more than five months in a hospital room. Try five weeks. I will tell you what. Try five days. As I have repeated often, but it warrants saying again…and succinctly: the staff kept me sane. But even with a great staff and care, the walls began to move. Toward me. I was going to become a mural that would be there forever. Okay, I know that was a little nuts. But that is how crazy you can get. I knew there were people around me who were having much longer stays. My heart went out to them. How were they going to do it? God, grant them mercy.

Here is what made things worse: unintended consequences. It worked this way. Almost every day, someone would come in and say, "Mr. Clews, it looks like you might be going home tomorrow. No promises, but…" I should capitalize the word "but." My hopes would get up with the first part of the sentence, and then…"but." The "but" seemed to be more relevant than any other word in the sentence. It turned out the next sentence had a worse word: "Surgery." I was going to have another surgery. The fluid had to go. One day, a doctor I had never met before came to my room. He was a very nice doctor with an easy manner. It should have made the bad news he came to deliver a little easier to take. He told me that another surgery was necessary. I just about lost it right there in my bed. "What? What the hell's left to operate on?"

He calmly explained that they wanted to do something that would, hopefully, once and for all solve the fluid buildup issue. As I understood it, they were going to place four tubes in my left rib cage that would allow fluid to drain from my body.

"Look, if it will solve this problem and get me out of here, you can put a blow hole in the top of my head."

The procedure, aka surgery, lasted somewhere between three and four hours. When, after some time in ICU, I was finally returned to my room, I had four tubes sticking out of my side. Four tubes, each one with a diameter about the size of a nickel, all draining fluid into a tank next to my bed. The tank had lines to measure the amount of fluid those tubes were draining from my body. Before I could go home, my side had to be tube-free. In the midst of all of this, there was a silver lining. I wasn't going to be seen in public with that lousy damn haircut.

*From the poem "If" by Rudyard Kipling

# Chapter 30
# Passing Homes Lit for Christmas

There were nights when I would wake up well after midnight. I would leave the room dark and look out my window toward a building somewhere near the hospital. With the Yuletide music playing in my room, I would stare at a lit Christmas tree in someone's apartment across the way.

Apparently, one night I must have pointed the scene out to Ashleigh. Shortly after that, she brought me a small, live pine tree in a pot. It had little lights already strung around it. She had a box with miniature balls for us to put on the tree. We spent some precious father/daughter time decorating that small Christmas tree, which then lived in my room for the rest of my stay. I would go to sleep listening to music, looking at my tree and, sometimes, singing carols to myself:

> *Silent night! Holy night!*
> *All is calm all is bright*
> *round yon virgin mother and child*
> *Holy infant so tender and mild*
> *sleep in heavenly peace!*

## PASSING HOMES LIT FOR CHRISTMAS

It was a tradition on Christmas Eve for my father to play the piano and sing this special Christmas hymn. He used to tell a story about World War I on Christmas Eve. As I recall, it went something like this. The fighting had stopped for the night. British soldiers were hunkered down in their trenches. From across Flanders Field, they heard German troops singing:

*Stille Nacht, heilige Nacht,*
*Alles schläft; einsam wacht*
*Nur das traute hochheilige Paar.*
*Holder Knabe im lockigen Haar,*
*Schlaf in himmlischer Ruh!*
*Schlaf in himmlischer Ruh!*

From their own trenches, the British replied:

*Silent night! Holy night!*
*Shepherds quake at the sight*
*glories stream from heaven afar*
*heavenly hosts sing Alleluia*
*Christ the Savior is born!*

The news on my surgery was that it was successful. The tube system was working. Fluid from my body was dripping into that clear container that measured the exited villain of the piece. The nurses measured it every day. Each time the container showed less fluid, they would remove a tube from my side. We knew that when the fluid was gone, so was Vince...to home, that is.

Carol and the transplant coordinator began to prepare us for the transition home, setting a plan for the massive amount of medications I was going to be taking to keep my body from rejecting the new heart. She told us about the kind of daily schedule of doses I would need to follow as a transplant patient for the rest of my life. She was very nice and thorough. And insistent that I listen. She would talk right over the TV. It became clear very quickly that she did not understand the importance of hearing dialogue to follow a story line.

The doctor was visiting one day when he decided that the first tube could come out. Of course, they had to pull it out. I braced myself, and *plup—numero uno* was out. Number two came out a little prematurely when I got up to go to the bathroom and stepped on it. Pow! It was out. Excitement grew. Honestly, I thought about stepping on the other two and getting the hell out of Dodge. But I was cautioned to be more respectful of the program, so I was. I watched the lines measuring the fluid in the container like a hawk measuring its prey. So did the doctor. It took about another week, and then number three was taken out. Somewhere around the thirteenth or fourteenth of December, the last tube was removed. I was ready to go, but the doctor wanted to observe me for a few more days before he would make a final decision. Several times we were told, "Tomorrow looks like the day." Tomorrow came and went. "Maybe tomorrow." Nope, not that one. Nor the next tomorrow, either. "What we've got here is a failure to communicate."

One day, "tomorrow" came. On December 19, 2013, after nearly six months in the hospital, Dr. Feller issued my release. I called Carol. "Honey, it's me. Can you be here around noon?"

"Is something wrong? Please, Vince, tell me nothing has happened."

"I'm coming home."

"What? Oh, my God! Oh, honey. I'm so happy for you. For us. This is it!"

"Yep. This is it."

Carol arrived more quickly than a law-abiding, safe driver should have. That was fine with me. I had done little preparation for my exit. Carol got right to work. She packed my things in plastic bags and carry-on bags. After nearly six months of living there, it was like moving out of an apartment. I left some things, like my mini-fridge. I kept the unique plant that a client, Brightline, sent and that had lived in my room with me for months. Carol was scrambling to get us out. The place was a zoo. And I could not help. She even had to help me get dressed. It turned out that Dr. Feller's earlier statement that I would be skinny when I left was true. My tighty-whiteys looked like boxers on me. I was so happy. Finally, my weight was not an issue in my life. I was skinny!

There was a flow of staff coming and doing things to me I cannot mention here. Mostly because I have no idea what they were. All I knew was, every time they left, they would say how happy they were for me. The nurses and the techs—everyone we met who could—came to say goodbye. How in the world do you make a family out of a hospital staff? You do not. They do. And they had.

I had always heard the phrase, "Parting is such sweet sorrow." So this is what it meant.

Carol loaded everything into the car. And, finally, I was wheeled to the front door and, subsequently, helped into the front seat by one of the guys from valet parking. He called me by name. "I'll just give you a hand here, Mr. Clews." He did not know me, but like all the front-area staff, they knew Mrs. Clews. And, just as everyone does who gets to know her, they liked her. I was, once again, the beneficiary. Just after eight o'clock, the car pulled away from my home away from home.

As we drove down one of Baltimore's streets, I began calling people to share the news. "Guess where I am? In the car headed home." I did not even notice the potholes and bumps in the street. This was a flight on a magic carpet. I stayed awake long enough to see the honky-tonks, strip clubs, and the once-famous Gayety Theater, all that I frequented as a young school boy and college student. I fell in love with Kelly Barton and Her Magic Lamp there. As we turned onto the expressway that supplies many people with their main exit from the city, I finally felt that I was really on my way home. I could not wait to see all the sights I had not seen in months. I fell asleep. Even the thrill of the ride home could not overcome the exhaustion from all I had been through.

When I awoke, we were on old familiar Nicodemus Road, just about a mile and a half from home. As we passed houses along the road, I could see the holiday season in the windows. I cracked the car window so I could smell the crisp air of winter. I breathed in the aroma of wood-burning in fireplaces. I saw the sky, the moon, and the stars. I think I recall one star being especially bright. Yes, Christmas really was here. And I was well enough to be home for it. "Thank you, Lord."

Now we were approaching the house. I could feel my new heart racing. It had already adapted to its new home. We pulled into the driveway. Carol stopped outside the garage and walked around to help me out of the car and onto my walker. One slow step at a time. I wanted to run. Not really. The drugs had not been that hallucinogenic. Finally, we were at the front door. I recalled a time decades ago when my father was coming home from an extended hospital stay. As he started up the steps to the front door, he began to weep. As I stepped up to the door, I knew why he had that reaction to the moment. Tears began to well. I stopped. It was overwhelming. I waited. Then Carol opened the door, and we walked in. I looked into the living room. The Christmas tree was fully decorated and lit. We walked into the family room, and Carol helped me slip gently into my old chair.

An anonymous writer wrote, "Home is where the heart is." Welcome home, new friend.

*THE BEGINNING*

# Postscript

As I am finishing this book, I am celebrating my seventh year as a heart transplant patient. Seven years. The average life expectancy for a transplant patient varies according to the source of the information. The consensus seems to be between five and twenty years. I have broken through the first threshold.

My heart (the heart I was given) has remained strong. So strong that I no longer require regular biopsies. That is a long way from once a month after I first came home. The biopsy visits turned into the same kind of family affair as my time in the hospital. And, just as during my stay, the staff became individuals Carol and I learned to love. Too many people were too good to mention names for fear of forgetting one. To each one, thank you for making me a member of your family. I do have to tell Gloria, the first person to greet us on each visit, which she does like a loving cousin, "You are a pip. God bless you."

Being home was both exhilarating and frightening. Carol took two weeks off work to stay with me. When she returned to her job, our friend, Ron Esposito, stayed with me for two weeks. Michael, Ashleigh, Patrick, and Griff continued to provide rides to my doctors' appointments and generally "dote on me/us." After Ron left, Marcia and Ernie came up to stay with me. Carter often filled in any gaps.

As Ralph and AJ had throughout all the months prior to my hospitalization, they were there daily to provide for any needs I could not attend to myself. And they often brought dinner so Carol did not have to come home and cook. The Frances are dictionary definitions of "friends." I am blessed to have such extraordinary friends and consider them family.

Because I left the hospital fairly well-rehabilitated, I was able to get up the stairs, back in my bedroom, and into our bed. Actually, the bed could have been a cardboard box under the expressway, just as long as Carol was in it with me. And I was in it with her.

At last, things were getting back to normal. Or so it seemed. That is, until one day when I felt a sudden pain in my side, more toward the back. And another, and almost instantly another. With each strike, the pain lasted longer until it was one extensive, very bad, pain. Carol witnessed this and spared no time in calling an ambulance. I was all for it this time. It turned out that it was my gallbladder. The next day, I had emergency surgery. Another visit to my friends in the cardiac unit. Once a heart patient, always a heart patient.

You may recall my disappointment at not being able to go to an Orioles game during my hospitalization. My friend, Natalie Seltz, who is a huge baseball fan, promised to take me to the Orioles 2014 opening day if I was well enough in time to make it. I was, and she did. Earlier, for my first post-transplant Christmas, my son, Chris, had given me a

T-shirt. It read "Team Tin Man." I wore it to the ball game.

On a Sunday near the end of March 2014, I finally returned to church and, once again, took communion with Carol. As Fr. Drake saw me approach the altar, he uncharacteristically threw his fist in the air. I love that guy. Soon after my return to church, Fr. Drake asked me to speak. It was an honor to accept. I talked about my (our) journey, my healing, and the role faith and prayer played in my healing. Dr. Porterfield was there, which was very nice. The service was one week before the O's Opening Day. I showed the ticket Natalie gave me just to demonstrate how well I was. In truth, Carol should have been the one speaking. I remind people all the time, it was Carol whose faith and strength were the constants that held everything together throughout our journey.

My rehab plan continued at home, exercising with light weights. I walked three miles every day. There was no required diet, but Carol made sure we ate like there was one. Things were moving along well until January 2014, I tripped and fell, fracturing my right hip. Back to surgery. Screws in my hip. The fracture was not good enough. In August 2015, I fell again, this time walking the dog. That time, I broke my left hip. The hip had to be replaced. Another hospital stay and rehab. Once again, Ralph and AJ were there for me and the dog every day. Of course, they were also there for Carol, as was Mike.

So now I had had two total knee replacements, screws in my right hip (which were subsequently taken out), and a replaced left hip. You would think

## POSTSCRIPT

I would be a pretty crippled-up fellow. On the contrary, I was actually pretty fit. Until the summer of 2017. I fell again. No trip. I was just walking when my right leg went out from under me and I fell. The fall was the result of an exposed nerve on a bulging disc in my back. Once again, I had to go under the knife. During recovery I was stuck on the second floor of our home. Ralph and AJ came over every day to bring my lunch upstairs to me and let Checkers out. The dog loves them like family. And rightly so.

Throughout all these post-transplant surgeries, I was the recipient of wonderful rehabilitation at the local Pivot Rehabilitation Center. I have been there so often that Sheryl Kohls, my primary therapist, has named one of the exercise tables after me. And, become a friend. I often say to people, "I am the healthiest broken man you know. I have the heart of the Tin Man. Sadly, I have the body of the Straw Man."

My heart has been through quite a bit since the transplant. It has never caused a minute of doubt. I guess this is what happens when your cardiologist makes sure you are given the "exactly right" heart.

# Appendix

Here are the documents contained in this appendix:

1. The letter Carol sent to Vice President Richard Cheney

2. Three letters from the University of Maryland Medical Center informing me of my status on the heart and kidney transplant lists. There were many others. Note that the letter dated October 25, 2013, finally removes me from the kidney list, two days before a heart was found for my transplant. (Whew!)

3. My official surgery report. It has been reformatted into book form for easier reading.

4. Sampling of the Scripture verses given to me by Fr. David Drake, which I include for comfort for others in difficult times.

APPENDIX

# The Letter Carol Sent to Dick Cheney, April 10, 2013

April 10, 2013

Vice President Richard Cheney
American Enterprise Institute for Public Policy Research
1150 Seventeenth Street, N.W.
Washington, D.C. 20036

Dear Mr. Cheney,

    I am writing to you because I have a favor to ask of you. I totally understand that this is coming out of nowhere, and I've no business making assumptions, but knowing what you've been through medically, I feel led to ask for your help.
    My husband, Vince Clews, was diagnosed about seven years ago with severe heart disease and has been in and out of the hospital battling this ever since.
    He is currently on the waiting list at University of Maryland Hospital for a heart (also kidney) transplant. He's in the hospital now, and has been for

six weeks, for a number of reasons, but mostly for fluid retention. I'm sure you are familiar with that and the myriad of ailments that accompany severe heart failure. I think it's fair to say that he is becoming discouraged, to say the least.

He's 69 years old. He's a talented writer with a great wit. He's a terrific husband and father and is a passionate lover of life in general. Truly, to know him is to love him. AND, by the way, he's a dyed-in-the-wool conservative and was never happier politically than when you and President Bush were in the White House.

I would like you to contact him to offer him some encouragement. I know that's asking a lot, but this has been going on for a while, and of course it could conceivably go on for a lot longer. I think a note from you would mean the world to him.

His home information is:
Vince Clews
1205 Nicodemus Road
Reisterstown, Maryland 21136
Cell phone: (410) xxx-xxxx

I appreciate your help, Mr. Cheney!

With respect and gratitude,
Carol Clews

# APPENDIX

# Letter from UMMC, March 6, 2013

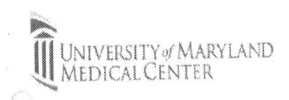

**UNIVERSITY of MARYLAND MEDICAL CENTER**

Cardiac Surgery
Heart and Lung Transplantation

29 S. Greene Street, Room 430
Baltimore, MD 21201
410-328-2854 | 443-462-3045 FAX

March 6, 2013

Mr. William Clews
1205 Nicodmeus Road
Reisterstown, MD 21136

Dear Mr. Clews:

We would like to inform you that your status on the UNOS heart transplant waiting list has changed. As of Thursday, March 28, 2013, you are inactive on the heart and kidney transplant list due to your recent infection.

You will receive more information regarding your status from your transplant physician and coordinator.

The United Network for Organ Sharing provides a toll-free patient services line to help transplant candidates, recipients and family members understand organ allocation practices and transplantation data. **Please see the attached letter for detailed information from the United Network for Organ Sharing.** You may also call this number to discuss a problem you may be experiencing with your transplant center or the transplantation system in general. The toll-free patient services line number is 1-888-894-6361.

If you have any questions, please feel free to call our office at (410) 328-2864.

Sincerely,

Andrea Banworth, RN
Heart Transplant Coordinator
CardioThoracic Transplantation

Enclosure

cc: Dr. Stuart Russell

Member of the University of Maryland Medical System
Affiliated with the University of Maryland School of Medicine

MY HEART TRANSPLANT FOR YOUR AMUSEMENT

# Letter from UMMC, March 25, 2013

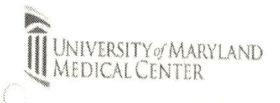

**UNIVERSITY of MARYLAND MEDICAL CENTER**

Cardiac Surgery
Heart and Lung Transplantation

29 S. Greene Street, Room 430
Baltimore, MD 21201
410-328-2864 | 443-462-3045 FAX

March 25, 2013

Mr. William Clews
1205 Nicodmeus Road
Reisterstown, MD 21136

Dear Mr. Clews:

We would like to inform you that your status on the UNOS heart transplant waiting list has changed. As of Monday, March 25, 2013, you are, once again, active on the heart transplant list as a status 1B and active on the kidney transplant list.

You will receive more information regarding your status from your transplant physician and coordinator.

The United Network for Organ Sharing provides a toll-free patient services line to help transplant candidates, recipients and family members understand organ allocation practices and transplantation data. **Please see the attached letter for detailed information from the United Network for Organ Sharing.** You may also call this number to discuss a problem you may be experiencing with your transplant center or the transplantation system in general. The toll-free patient services line number is 1-888-894-6361.

If you have any questions, please feel free to call our office at (410) 328-2864.

Sincerely,

*Andrea Banworth, RN*
Andrea Banworth, RN
Heart Transplant Coordinator
CardioThoracic Transplantation

Enclosure

cc. Dr. Stuart Russell

---

Member of the University of Maryland Medical System
Affiliated with the University of Maryland School of Medicine

APPENDIX

# Letter from UMMC, October 23, 2013

**UNIVERSITY of MARYLAND MEDICAL CENTER**

Cardiac Surgery
Heart and Lung Transplantation

29 S. Greene Street, Room 430
Baltimore, MD 21201
410-328-2864   443-462-5045 FAX

October 23, 2012

Mr. William Clews
1205 Nicodemus Road
Reisterstown, MD 21136

Dear Mr. Clews:

This letter is to inform you of your official listing on Kidney UNOS/OPTN National Transplant Waiting List, effective Friday, October 19, 2012 with the University of Maryland Medical Center being your designated Transplant Center. As you were previously informed, your status on the Heart Transplant Waiting list was upgraded to status 1B effective Wednesday, October 17, 2012.

Successful heart/kidney transplantation requires a partnership with the transplant team, the referring physician, and most importantly, you, the patient. To remain active on the heart transplant waiting list, we expect that you will:

- *Abstain from all alcohol and other substances of abuse*
- *Identify a significant other that will be your primary support during your hospitalization and recovery*
- *Demonstrate adherence to medical recommendations by:*
    - *Keeping your appointments*
    - *Taking your medications as prescribed*
    - *Following through with physician recommendations*
    - *Getting all necessary tests done in a timely fashion.*

**FAILURE TO COMPLY WITH THE ABOVE EXPECTATIONS MAY RESULT IN YOUR REMOVAL FROM THE TRANSPLANT WAITING LIST.**

The United Network for Organ Sharing provides a toll-free patient services line to help transplant candidates, recipients and family members understand organ allocation practices and transplantation data. **Please see the attached letter for detailed information from the United Network for Organ Sharing.** You may also call this number to discuss a problem you may be experiencing with your transplant center or the transplantation system in general. The toll-free patient services line number is 1-888-894-6361.

---

Member of the University of Maryland Medical System
Affiliated with the University of Maryland School of Medicine

Mr. William Clews
October 23, 2012
Page 2

You will receive more information regarding your status from your transplant physician and coordinator.

If you have any questions, please feel free to call our office at 410-328-2864.

Sincerely,

*Andrea Banworth, RN*
Andrea Banworth, RN
Heart Transplant Coordinator
CardioThoracic Transplantation

Enclosure

cc: Charles Cangro, MD
    Stuart Russell, MD
    John Sperati, MD

APPENDIX

# Letter from UMMC, October 25, 2013

**UNIVERSITY of MARYLAND MEDICAL CENTER**

Cardiac Surgery
Heart and Lung Transplantation

29 S. Greene Street, Room 430
Baltimore, MD 21201
410-328-2864 | 443-462-3045 FAX

October 25, 2013

Mr. William Clews
1205 Nicodemus Road
Reisterstown, MD 21136

Dear Mr. Clews:

We would like to inform you that your status on the UNOS kidney transplant waiting list has changed. As of October 24, 2013 you have been removed from the kidney transplant list. It has been determined that you do not need a kidney transplant at this time.

You will receive more information regarding your status from your transplant physician and coordinator.

The United Network for Organ Sharing provides a toll-free patient services line to help transplant candidates, recipients and family members understand organ allocation practices and transplantation data. **Please see the attached letter for detailed information from the United Network for Organ Sharing.** You may also call this number to discuss a problem you may be experiencing with your transplant center or the transplantation system in general. The toll-free patient services line number is 1-888-894-6361.

If you have any questions, please feel free to call our office at (410) 328-2864.

Sincerely,

Erika D. Feller, MD
Assistant Professor of Medicine
Medical Director, Heart Transplantation

Whitney Amereihn, RN
Heart Transplant Coordinator

Enclosure

---
Member of the University of Maryland Medical System
Affiliated with the University of Maryland School of Medicine

MY HEART TRANSPLANT FOR YOUR AMUSEMENT

# Surgery Notes from UMMC, December 19, 2013

Facility: UNIVERSITY OF MARYLAND MEDICAL CENTER
110 South Paca Street, 9th Floor
Baltimore MD 21201-1595
Notes Report

Clews, William
MRN: 0001979060, DOB: 9/5/1943, Sex: M
Adm: 6/30/2013, D/C: 12/19/2013

## Notes

**Procedures signed by Keshava Rajagopal at 10/29/13 1040**

| Author: Keshava Rajagopal | Service: (none) | Author Type: Physician |
|---|---|---|
| Filed: 10/29/13 1044 | Date of Service: 10/27/13 2235 | Status: Signed |
| Editor: Keshava Rajagopal (Physician) | | |

MRN: 1979060
PATIENT NAME: CLEWS, WILLIAM
DATE OF BIRTH: 09/05/43
GENDER: M
DATE OF PROCEDURE: 10/27/13
SURGEON: RAJAGOPAL, KESHAVA, M.D., PH.D.
CO-SURGEON: PHAM, SI, M.D.
FIRST ASSISTANT: WATKINS, AMELIA, M.D.
SERVICE: SCA - CARDIAC SURGERY

PREOPERATIVE DIAGNOSIS: End-stage heart disease, secondary to restrictive/infiltrative cardiomyopathy due to amyloidosis.

POSTOPERATIVE DIAGNOSIS: End-stage heart disease, secondary to restrictive/infiltrative cardiomyopathy due to amyloidosis.

OPERATIVE PROCEDURE:
1. Back-table preparation of cardiac allograft.
2. Ligation of left atrial appendage.
3. Orthotopic cardiac transplantation via bicaval technique.
4. Removal of AICD generator and leads.

ANESTHESIA: General endotracheal.

ANESTHESIOLOGIST:

CARDIOPULMONARY BYPASS TIME: 207 minutes.

ALLOGRAFT ISCHEMIC TIME: 264 minutes.

INTRAVENOUS FLUIDS:
1. 1500 mL Cell Saver.
2. 9 units packed red blood cells, 4 units platelets, 8 units fresh frozen plasma, and 2 units cryoprecipitate.

ESTIMATED BLOOD LOSS: See anesthesia/perfusion records.

DRAINS:
1. Mediastinum: 32-French straight tube thoracostomy, 19-French Blake drains x2.
2. Bilateral pleural spaces: 32-French right angle chest tube, 1 in each pleural space.

SPECIMENS: Native heart, to Pathology.

FINDINGS: Satisfactory completion noninvasive/invasive physiological studies/data.

# APPENDIX

Facility: UNIVERSITY OF MARYLAND MEDICAL CENTER  Clews, William
110 South Paca Street, 9th Floor  MRN: 0001979060, DOB: 9/5/1943, Sex: M
Baltimore MD 21201-1595  Adm: 6/30/2013, D/C: 12/19/2013
Notes Report

**Procedures signed by Keshava Rajagopal at 10/29/13 1040 (continued)**

COMPLICATIONS: None immediate.

DISPOSITION: Adequate and stable, to Cardiac Surgical Intensive Care Unit.

1. Milrinone infusion at 0.25 mcg/kg per minute, epinephrine infusion at 0.05 mcg/kg per minute, norepinephrine infusion at 10 mcg/minute, vasopressin infusion at 0.06 units/minute.
2. Invasively mechanically ventilated at relatively standard settings; inhaled nitric oxide 40 parts per million.

INDICATIONS: Mr. Clews is a 70-year-old man with end-stage heart disease secondary to restrictive/infiltrative cardiomyopathy due to amyloidosis. He underwent thorough diagnostic evaluation, and was deemed a suitable candidate for orthotopic heart transplantation. A good quality candidate allograft became available, and the patient was taken to the operating room for planned orthotopic heart transplantation.

PROCEDURE: After informed consent was obtained, the patient was taken to the operating room, placed in supine position on operating table. Intravenous sedatives and anesthetics were administered, once an adequate level of sedation had been achieved, the patient was endotracheally intubated. Invasive hemodynamic monitoring lines, comprised of a right brachial arterial catheter, and a right internal jugular venous introducer sheath through which a pulmonary arterial catheter was initially advanced into the main pulmonary artery and subsequently withdrawn into the right internal jugular vein, were placed by the Cardiac Anesthesiology Team. A transesophageal echocardiography probe was placed by the Cardiac Anesthesiology Team.

Once these procedures were complete, the operative field was prepared and draped in the standard sterile fashion. A surgical time-out was performed.

Next, median sternotomy was undertaken in the standard fashion, using a #10 blade scalpel for the skin, with electrocautery for the superficial and deep subcutaneous tissues. Invasive mechanical ventilation was transiently interrupted, the sternum was divided in the midline using a saw. Sternal edge hemostasis was achieved using topical of application of vancomycin paste and electrocautery. A Morris retractor was placed, and the pericardium was opened. Pericardial stay sutures were placed and affixed to the skin.

Next, the patient was systemically anticoagulated with heparin, 300 units/kg administered as an intravenous bolus dose. Attention was next paid to cannulation for an institution of cardiopulmonary bypass. Attention was first paid to systemic arterial/ascending thoracic aortic cannulation. Two rhombus shaped 3-0 Ethibond pursestring cannulation sutures were placed on the anterior surface of the distal ascending thoracic aorta, with the inner set nonpledgeted and the outer set doubly pledgeted at the 3 and 9 o'clock positions, and these were secured using

Printed on 4/23/19 12:34 PM

# MY HEART TRANSPLANT FOR YOUR AMUSEMENT

Facility: UNIVERSITY OF MARYLAND MEDICAL CENTER  Clews, William
110 South Paca Street, 9th Floor   MRN: 0001979060, DOB: 9/5/1943, Sex: M
Baltimore MD 21201-1595   Adm: 6/30/2013, D/C: 12/19/2013
Notes Report

## Procedures signed by Keshava Rajagopal at 10/29/13 1040 (continued)

Rommel devices. An appropriate systemic arterial blood pressure for ascending thoracic aortic cannulation was ensured. The adventitia in the region of ascending thoracic aorta circumscribed by the pursestring cannulation sutures was incised using Metzenbaum scissors. Next, a #11 blade scalpel was used to create a stab aortotomy in the region of aorta circumscribed by the pursestring cannulation sutures. Quickly, a 22-French Medtronic EOPA systemic arterial cannula was introduced into the aortotomy, and advanced 2.5 cm. The Rommel devices securing the cannulation sutures were tightened, and in turn secured to the cannula. The introducer for the ascending thoracic aortic cannula was withdrawn slowly, and the free end of the cannula was clamped using a tubing clamp. A gasless connection was made to the systemic arterial line of the cardiopulmonary bypass circuit. The tubing clamp on the ascending thoracic aortic cannula was removed, and once a therapeutic activated clotting time was achieved, a test bolus of 100 mL of priming volume was administered antegrade via the cardiopulmonary bypass circuit through the ascending thoracic aortic cannula. This was well-tolerated without issue. Next, attention was paid to systemic venous cannulation.
Attention was first paid to superior vena caval cannulation. A rhombus shaped nonpledgeted 2-0 Ethibond pursestring cannulation suture was placed in the anterior surface of the superior vena cava and secured using the Rommel device. A #11 blade scalpel was used to create a stab superior vena cavotomy in the region of the superior vena cava circumscribed by the pursestring cannulation suture. This was gently dilated using a tonsil clamp. Attempts were made to pass a 28-French Medtronic flexible blunt-tipped cannula and institute partial cardiopulmonary bypass through this cannula, but these were unsuccessful. Ultimately, a 24-French Medtronic metal-tipped right-angled cannula was introduced into the superior vena cavotomy, and advanced until the hub was flush. In the course of doing this, the cannulation site tore superiorly, and a 2nd pursestring cannulation suture was placed at the superior vena caval cannulation site. This was a rhombus shaped doubly pledgeted 4-0 Prolene suture, doubly pledgeted at the 12 and 6 o'clock positions. The superior vena caval cannula was connected to one of the limbs of the venous line of the cardiopulmonary bypass circuit. Partial cardiopulmonary bypass was initiated through the superior vena caval cannula, with initial maintenance of systemic normothermia. Attention was next paid to inferior vena caval cannulation. An hexagonal shaped 2-0 Ethibond nonpledgeted pursestring cannulation suture was placed on the anterior surface of the inferior vena cava, this secured using Rommel device. A #11 blade scalpel was used to create a stab inferior vena cavotomy, this was gently dilated using a tonsil clamp. Quickly, a 28-French Medtronic metal-tipped right-angled systemic venous cannula was introduced into the inferior vena cavotomy, and advanced until the hub was flush. The Rommel device securing the pursestring cannulation suture was tightened, and returned secured to the cannula. The inferior vena caval cannula was connected to the 2nd venous limb of the venous line of the cardiopulmonary bypass circuit, and total cardiopulmonary bypass via bicaval systemic venous cannulation was initiated. Mild systemic hypothermia to 32-degrees Centigrade was initiated. Invasive mechanical ventilation was continued throughout the cardiopulmonary bypass portion of the case at low tidal

Printed on: 4/23/19 12:34 PM

## APPENDIX

Facility: UNIVERSITY OF MARYLAND MEDICAL CENTER
110 South Paca Street, 9th Floor
Baltimore MD 21201-1595
Notes Report

Clews, William
MRN: 0001979060, DOB: 9/5/1943, Sex: M
Adm: 6/30/2013, D/C: 12/19/2013

### Procedures signed by Keshava Rajagopal at 10/29/13 1040 (continued)

volumes.

Next, the superior and inferior vena cavae were encircled using caval tapes, which were secured using Rommel devices. Next, cardiopulmonary bypass flow rates were transiently reduced, and the distal ascending thoracic aorta was cross clamped, at a location just proximal to the ascending thoracic aortic cannula. The native heart fibrillated, and attention was next paid to native recipient cardiectomy. The native heart was excised in the standard fashion. The ascending thoracic aorta was transected at the sinotubular junction. The main pulmonary artery was transected just distal to the pulmonary valve. An oblique right atriotomy was created, beginning of the right atrial appendage, and continuing inline with the right-sided atrioventricular groove through the coronary sinus. The fossa ovalis was incised sharply using a #11 blade scalpel. Attention was next paid to placement of a left ventricular vent catheter. A rhombus shaped 3-0 Ethibond pursestring cannulation suture, doubly pledgeted at the 12 and 6 o'clock positions, was placed in the anterior face of the right superior pulmonary vein and secured using Rommel device. A #11 blade scalpel was used to create a stab right superior pulmonary venotomy. 20-French Medtronic DLP vent catheter was introduced into the right superior pulmonary vein, and advanced until the tip passed into the left superior pulmonary vein. The recipient cardiectomy was completed. The operative field was flooded with CO2.

At this point, the donor heart arrived in the operating room, and was unpackaged. It appeared to be in excellent condition, without any evidence of structural injury or defect. The left atrial appendage was ligated using a 4-0 Prolene pursestring suture circumferentially around the base of the appendage and a 0 silk tie superficial to this. A dose of cold blood cardioplegia was administered antegrade via the ascending thoracic aorta of the donor cardiac allograft, 500 mL in volume. Attention was next paid to implantation of the donor cardiac allograft. Attention was first paid to creation of the left atrial anastomosis. An end-to-end recipient to donor left atrial anastomosis was created using 4-0 Prolene suture on an SH needle in continuous fashion, circumferentially. Towards the completion of this anastomosis, the left ventricular vent catheter was repositioned and advanced across the mitral valve such that the tip of the catheter resided within the donor cardiac allograft left ventricle. The left ventricular vent catheter was connected to one of the vent/cardiotomy suction lines of the cardiopulmonary bypass circuit. Next, attention was paid to creation of the ascending thoracic aortic anastomosis, which was to be performed in two-layer fashion. An additional dose of cold blood cardioplegia, 500 mL of volume, was administered antegrade via the ascending thoracic aorta. The recipient ascending thoracic aorta was trimmed to an appropriate length in a straight (no bevelling) fashion. The donor ascending thoracic aorta, which was somewhat smaller in circumference, was trimmed with a beveled angle, such that the bevel extended from superior to inferior with a superior overhang. Next, an end-to-end donor to recipient ascending thoracic aortic anastomosis was created using 4-0 Prolene suture on a BB-1 needle in continuous horizontal mattress

## MY HEART TRANSPLANT FOR YOUR AMUSEMENT

Facility: UNIVERSITY OF MARYLAND MEDICAL CENTER  Clews, William
110 South Paca Street, 9th Floor
Baltimore MD 21201-1595
MRN: 0001979060, DOB: 9/5/1943, Sex: M
Adm: 6/30/2013, D/C: 12/19/2013
Notes Report

### Procedures signed by Keshava Rajagopal at 10/29/13 1040 (continued)

fashion. A second layer of the donor-to-recipient ascending thoracic aortic anastomosis was created an end-to-end configuration using 4-0 Prolene suture on a BB-1 needle in continuous fashion circumferentially. During the creation of this anastomotic suture line, systemic rewarming was initiated. At the completion of this anastomosis, a 4-0 Prolene horizontal mattress suture, doubly pledgeted at the 12 and 6 o'clock positions, was placed on the anterior surface of the distal aspect of the donor ascending thoracic aorta, just proximal to the ascending thoracic aortic anastomosis. A needle-tipped antegrade cardioplegia/ascending aortic vent catheter was used to create a stab aortotomy in the region of aorta circumscribed by the horizontal mattress suture. The Rommel device securing the horizontal mattress suture was tightened, and in turn secured to the catheter. A dose of warm blood ("hotshot") cardioplegia, 500 mL in volume, was administered antegrade via the ascending thoracic aorta, with the ascending aortic vent open for the first 50 mL of infusion. Left ventricular venting was continued during this procedure, and left ventricular vent catheter return was not augmented, nor was there left ventricular distention, thus suggestive of the absence of aortic valve regurgitation. After completion of the administration of the dose of warm blood ("hotshot") cardioplegia, cardiopulmonary bypass flow rates were transiently reduced, an ascending thoracic aortic cross-clamp was released. The donor cardiac allograft resumed electrical activity in ventricular fibrillation, and a single defibrillation was required to achieve a junctional cardiac rhythm. Two right ventricular epicardial pacing wires were placed, exteriorized, and secured to the skin. VVI pacing at a rate of 90 was initiated.

Attention was next paid to creation of the main pulmonary arterial anastomosis. The donor and recipient main pulmonary arteries were trimmed in a straight fashion to an appropriate length. Next, an end-to-end donor to recipient main pulmonary arterial anastomosis was created using 5-0 Prolene suture in continuous fashion. Attention was next paid to creation of the inferior vena caval anastomosis. A flexible cardiotomy suction catheter was introduced into the free end of the superior vena cava of the donor cardiac allograft, and advanced into the coronary sinus. Next, an end-to-end recipient to donor inferior vena caval anastomosis was created using 4-0 Prolene suture in continuous fashion. After completion of this anastomosis, attention was paid to the superior vena caval anastomosis. A posterior slit was created in the donor superior vena cava. Next, an end-to-end recipient to donor superior vena caval enastomosis was created using 4-0 Prolene suture on an RB needle in continuous fashion. At the completion of this anastomosis, the caval tapes on the superior and inferior vena cavae were released.

The donor cardiac allograft appeared to function well while on full cardiopulmonary bypass. Attention was next paid to weaning/separation from cardiopulmonary bypass. Two right atrial epicardial pacing wires were placed, exteriorized, and secured to the skin. AAI pacing at a rate of 110 was initiated. Invasive mechanical ventilation at full levels was resumed. The aforementioned pharmacologic inotropic and

APPENDIX

Facility: UNIVERSITY OF MARYLAND MEDICAL CENTER
110 South Paca Street, 9th Floor
Baltimore MD 21201-1595
Notes Report

Clews, William
MRN: 0001979060, DOB: 9/5/1943, Sex: M
Adm: 6/30/2013, D/C: 12/19/2013

**Procedures signed by Keshava Rajagopal at 10/29/13 1040 (continued)**

present for the entirety of the case.

Dr. Pham and I were co-surgeons for this case. I opened the patient, placed the patient on cardiopulmonary bypass, placed the vent and cardioplegia catheters, and performed the implantation of the donor cardiac allograft with the exception of the inferior vena caval anastomosis. Dr. Pham performed the native cardiectomy, left atrial appendage ligation, and the inferior vena caval anastomosis, which was quite challenging. This operation also took an extended period of time, due to the severe sternal bleeding. The actual cardiac transplantation procedure took approximately 4 hours and 30 minutes, while the process of achieving superficial mediastinal hemostasis at the level of the sternum and superficial soft tissues, took a total of 3 hours and 30 minutes.

ATTENDING PHYSICIANS STATEMENT: I was present for the entire procedure.

----{ Related Clinicians: Docnum#: 4116422 }--------
PHAM, SI MAI { CC }
RAJAGOPAL, KESHAVA { DICT }
FELLER, ERIKA { REFER }
RAJAGOPAL, KESHAVA { SIGN 29-OCT-13 }

End of Dictated Report
This document has been read and signed. Please contact the medical records department for any questions regarding this document.

**END OF REPORT**

MY HEART TRANSPLANT FOR YOUR AMUSEMENT

# Notes from Dr. Lesjava Rajagopal, October 29, 2013

Procedures signed by Keshava Rajagopal at 10/29/131040
Author: Keshava Rajagopal   Service: (none)
Filed: 10/29/13 1044   Date of Service: 10/27/13
2235 Editor: Keshava Rajagopal (Physician)
Physician Status: Signed


MRN:          1979060
PATIENT NAME: CLEWS, WILLIAM
DATE OF BIRTH: 09/05/43
GENDER: M

DATE OF PROCEDURE: 10/27/13
SURGEON: RAJAGOPAL, KESHAVA, M.D., PH.D.
CO-SURGEON: PHAM, SI, M.D.
FIRST ASSISTANT: WATKINS, AMELIA, M.D.

SERVICE:    SCA- CARDIAC SURGERY

PREOPERATIVE DIAGNOSIS: End-stage heart disease, secondary to restrictive/infiltrative cardiomyopathy due to amyloidosis.

POSTOPERATIVE DIAGNOSIS: End-stage heart disease, secondary to restrictive/infiltrative cardiomyopathy due to amyloidosis.

OPERATIVE PROCEDURE:
1. Back-table preparation of cardiac allograft.
2. Ligation of left atrial appendage.

3. Orthotopic cardiac transplantation via bicaval technique.
4. Removal of AICD generator and leads.

ANESTHESIA: General endotracheal.
ANESTHESIOLOGIST:

CARDIOPULMONARY BYPASS TIME: 207 minutes. ALLOGRAFT ISCHEMIC TIME: 264 minutes.

INTRAVENOUS FLUIDS:
1. 1500 ml Cell Saver.
2. 9 units packed red blood cells, 4 units platelets, 8 units fresh frozen plasma, and 2 units cryoprecipitate.

ESTIMATED BLOOD LOSS: See anesthesia/perfusion records.

DRAINS:
1. Mediastinum: 32-French straight tube thoracostomy, 19-French Blake drains x2.
2. Bilateral pleural spaces: 32-French right angle chest tube, 1 in each pleural space.

SPECIMENS: Native heart, to Pathology.

FINDINGS: Satisfactory completion noninvasive/invasive physiological studies/data.

COMPLICATIONS: None immediate.

DISPOSITION: Adequate and stable, to Cardiac Surgical Intensive Care Unit.

1. Milrinone infusion at 0.25 mcg/kg per minute, epinephrine infusion. at 0.05 mcg/kg per minute, norepinephrine infusion at 10 mcg/minute, vasopressin infusion at 0.06 units/minute.
2. Invasively mechanically ventilated at relatively standard settings; inhaled nitric oxide 40 parts per million.

INDICATIONS: Mr. Clews is a 70-year-old man with end-stage heart disease secondary to restrictive/infiltrative cardiomyopathy due to amyloidosis. He underwent thorough diagnostic evaluation, and was deemed a suitable candidate for orthotopic heart transplantation. A good quality candidate allograft became available, and the patient was taken to the operating room for planned orthotopic heart transplantation.

PROCEDURE: After informed consent was obtained, the patient was taken to the operating room, placed in supine position on operating table.

Intravenous sedatives and anesthetics were administered, once an adequate level of sedation had been achieved, the patient was endotracheally intubated. Invasive hemodynamic monitoring lines, comprised of a right brachial arterial catheter, and a right internal jugular venous introducer sheath through which a pulmonary arterial catheter was initially advanced into the main pulmonary artery and subsequently withdrawn into the right internal jugular vein, were placed by the Cardiac Anesthesiology Team. A transesophageal echo-cardiography probe was placed by the Cardiac Anesthesiology Team.

# APPENDIX

Once these procedures were complete, the operative field was prepared and draped in the standard sterile fashion. A surgical time-out was performed.

Next, median sternotomy was undertaken in the standard fashion, using a #10 blade scalpel for the skin, with electrocautery for the superficial and deep subcutaneous tissues. Invasive mechanical venti-lation was transiently interrupted, the sternum was divided in the midline using a saw. Sternal edge hemostasis was achieved using topical of application of vancomycin paste and electrocautery. A Morris retractor was placed, and the pericardium was opened. Pericardial stay sutures were placed and affixed to the skin.

Next, the patient was systemically anticoagulated with heparin, 300 units/kg administered as an intravenous bolus dose. Attention was next paid to cannulation for an institution of cardiopulmonary bypass.

Attention was first paid to systemic arterial/ascending thoracic aortic cannulation. Two rhombus shaped 3-0 Ethibond pursestring cannulation sutures were placed on the anterior surface of the distal ascending thoracic aorta, with the inner set nonpledgeted and the outer set doubly pledgeted at the 3 and 9 o'clock positions, and these were secured using Rommel devices. An appropriate systemic arterial blood pressure for ascending thoracic aortic cannulation was ensured. The adventitia in the region of ascending thoracic aorta circumscribed by the pursestring cannulation sutures was incised using Metzenbaum scissors. Next, a #11 blade scalpel was used to create a stab aortotomy in the region of aorta circumscribed by the pursestring cannulation sutures. Quickly, a 22-French Medtronic EOPA systemic arterial cannula was introduced into the aortotomy, and advanced 2.5 cm. The Rommel devices securing the cannulation sutures were tightened, and in turn secured to the cannula. The introducer for the ascending thoracic aortic cannula was withdrawn slowly, and the free end of the cannula was clamped using a tubing clamp. A gasless connection was made to the systemic arterial line of the cardiopulmonary bypass circuit. The tubing clamp on the ascending thoracic aortic cannula was removed, and once a therapeutic activated clotting time was achieved, a test bolus of 100 ml of priming volume was administered antegrade via the cardiopulmonary bypass circuit through the ascending thoracic aortic cannula. This was well-tolerated without issue. Next, attention was paid to systemic venous cannulation.

Attention was first paid to superior vena caval cannulation. A rhombus shaped nonpledgeted 2-0 Ethibond pursestring cannulation suture was placed in the anterior surface of the superior vena cava and secured using the Rommel device. A #11 blade scalpel was used to create a stab superior vena cavotomy in the region of the superior vena cava circumscribed by the pursestring cannulation suture. This was gently dilated using a tonsil clamp. Attempts were made to pass a 28-French Medtronic flexible blunt-tipped cannula and institute partial cardiopulmonary bypass through this cannula, but these were unsuccessful. Ultimately, a 24-French Medtronic metal-tipped right-angled cannula was introduced into the superior vena cavotomy, and advanced until the hub was flush. In the course of doing this, the cannulation site tore superiorly, and a 2nd pursestring cannulation suture was placed at the superior vena caval cannulation site. This was a rhombus shaped doubly pledgeted 4-0 Prolene suture, doubly pledgeted at the 12 and 6 o'clock positions. The superior vena caval cannula was connected to one of the limbs of the venous line of the cardiopulmonary bypass circuit. Partial cardiopulmonary bypass was initiated through the superior vena caval cannula, with initial maintenance of systemic normothermia. Attention was next paid to inferior vena caval cannulation. An hexagonal shaped 2-0 Ethibond nonpledgeted pursestring cannulation suture was placed on the anterior surface of the inferior vena cava, this secured using Rommel device. A #11 blade scalpel was used to create a stab inferior vena cavotomy, this was gently dilated using a tonsil clamp. Quickly, a 28-French Medtronic metal-tipped right-angled systemic venous cannula was introduced into the inferior vena cavotomy, and advanced until the hub was flush. The Rommel device securing the pursestring cannulation suture was tightened, and returned secured to the cannula. The inferior vena caval cannula was connected to the 2nd venous limb of the venous line of the cardiopulmonary bypass circuit, and total cardiopulmonary bypass via bicaval systemic venous cannulation was initiated. Mild systemic hypo-thermia to 32-degrees Centigrade was initiated. Invasive mechanical ventilation was continued throughout the cardiopulmonary bypass portion of the case at low tidal volumes.

Next, the superior and inferior vena cavae were encircled using caval tapes, which were secured using Rommel devices. Next, cardiopulmonary bypass flow rates were transiently reduced, and the distal ascending thoracic aorta was cross clamped, at a

## MY HEART TRANSPLANT FOR YOUR AMUSEMENT

location just proximal to the ascending thoracic aortic cannula. The native heart fibrillated, and attention was next paid to native recipient cardiectomy. The native heart was excised in the standard fashion. The ascending thoracic aorta was transected at the sinotubular junction. The main pulmonary artery was transected just distal to the pulmonary valve. An oblique right atriotomy was created, beginning of the right atrial appendage, and continuing inline with the right-sided atrioventricular groove through the coronary sinus. The fossa ovalis was incised sharply using a #11 blade scalpel. Attention was next paid to placement of a left ventricular vent catheter. A rhombus shaped 3-0 Ethibond pursestring cannulation suture, doubly pledgeted at the 12 and 6 o'clock positions, was placed in the anterior surface of the right superior pulmonary vein and secured using Rommel device. A #11 blade scalpel was used to create a stab right superior pulmonary venotomy. 20-French Medtronic DlP vent catheter was introduced into the right superior pulmonary vein, and advanced until the tip passed into the left superior pulmonary vein.

The recipient cardiectomy was completed. The operative field was flooded with $CO_2$.

At this point, the donor heart arrived in the operating room, and was unpackaged. It appeared to be in excellent condition, without any evidence of structural injury or defect. The left atrial appendage was ligated using a 4-0 Prolene pursestring suture circumferentially around the base of the appendage and a O silk tie superficial to this. A dose of cold blood cardioplegia was administered antegrade via the ascending thoracic aorta of the donor cardiac allograft, 500 ml in volume.

Attention was next paid to implantation of the donor cardiac allograft. Attention was first paid to creation of the left atrial anastomosis. An end-to-end recipient to donor left atrial anastomosis was created using 4-0 Prolene suture on an SH needle in continuous fashion, circumferentially. Towards the completion of this anastomosis, the left ventricular vent catheter was repositioned and advanced across the mitral valve such that the tip of the catheter resided within the donor cardiac allograft left ventricle. The left ventricular vent catheter was connected to one of the vent/cardiotomy suction lines of the cardiopulmonary bypass circuit. Next, attention was paid to creation of the ascending thoracic aortic anastomosis, which was to be performed in two-layer fashion. An additional dose of cold blood cardioplegia, 500 ml of volume, was administered antegrade via the ascending thoracic aorta. The recipient ascending thoracic aorta was trimmed to an appropriate length in a straight (no bevelling) fashion. The donor ascending thoracic aorta, which was somewhat smaller in circumference, was trimmed with a beveled angle, such that the bevel extended from superior to inferior with a superior overhang. Next, an end-to-end donor to recipient ascending thoracic aortic anastomosis was created using 4-0 Prolene suture on a BB-1 needle in continuous horizontal mattress fashion. A second layer of the donor-to-recipient ascending thoracic aortic anastomosis was created an end-to-end configuration using 4-0 Prolene suture on a BB-1 needle in continuous fashion circumferentially. During the creation of this anastomotic suture line, systemic rewarming was initiated. At the completion of this anastomosis, a 4-0 Prolene horizontal mattress suture, doubly pledgeted at the 12 and 6 o'clock positions, was placed on the anterior surface of the distal aspect of the donor ascending thoracic aorta, just proximal to the ascending thoracic aortic anastomosis.

A needle-tipped antegrade cardioplegia/ascending aortic vent catheter was used to create a stab aortotomy in the region of aorta circumscribed by the horizontal mattress suture. The Rommel device securing the horizontal mattress suture was tightened, and in turn secured to the catheter. A dose of warm blood ("hotshot") cardioplegia, 500 ml in volume, was administered antegrade via the ascending thoracic aorta, with the ascending aortic vent open for the first 50 ml of infusion. Left ventricular venting was continued during this procedure, and left ventricular vent catheter return was not augmented, nor was there left ventricular distention, thus suggestive of the absence of aortic valve regurgitation. After completion of the administration of the dose of warm blood ("hotshot") cardioplegia, cardiopulmonary bypass flow rates were transiently reduced, an ascending thoracic aortic cross-clamp was released. The donor cardiac allograft resumed electrical activity in ventricular fibrillation, and a single defibrillation was required to achieve a junctional cardiac rhythm. Two right ventricular epicardial pacing wires were placed, exteriorized, and secured to the skin. WI pacing at a rate of 90 was initiated.

Attention was next paid to creation of the main pulmonary arterial anastomosis. The donor and recipient main pulmonary arteries were trimmed in a straight fashion to an appropriate length. Next, an end-to-end donor to recipient main pulmonary arterial anastomosis was created using 5-0 Prolene suture in continuous fashion. Attention was next paid to creation of the inferior vena caval anastomosis. A flexible cardiotomy suction catheter was introduced into the free end of the superior vena cava of the donor cardiac allograft, and advanced into the coronary sinus. Next, an end-to-end recipient to donor inferior vena caval anastomosis was created using 4-0 Prolene suture in continuous fashion. After completion of this anastomosis, attention was paid to the superior vena caval anastomosis. A posterior slit was created in the donor superior vena cava. Next, an end-to-end recipient to donor superior vena caval anastomosis was created using 4-0 Prolene suture on an RB needle in continuous fashion. At the completion of this anastomosis, the caval tapes on the superior and inferior vena cavae were released.

The donor cardiac allograft appeared to function well while on full cardiopulmonary bypass. Attention was next paid to weaning/separation from cardio-pulmonary bypass. Two right atrial epicardial pacing wires were placed, exteriorized, and secured to the skin. AAI pacing at a rate of 110 was initiated. Invasive mechanical ventilation at full levels was resumed. The aforementioned pharmacologic inotropic and vasoactive support was initiated. Next, volume was translocated from the cardiopulmonary bypass circuit to the patient, and cardiopulmonary bypass flow rates were slowly/iteratively weaned, until cardiopulmonary bypass was successfully discontinued without issue. Hemostasis within the mediastinum required the placement of 3 anastomotic repair sutures, 1 on the left posterior aspect of the left atrial anastomosis (4-0 Prolene doubly pledgeted horizontal mattress suture), 1 on the right anterior aspect of the main pulmonary arterial anastomosis, which appeared to be vigorous needle hole bleeding (5-0 Prolene nonpledgeted horizontal mattress suture). The last repair suture was in the anterior surface of the inferior vena cava, slightly leftward in location, in the vicinity of the coronary sinus. This was carefully repaired using a doubly pledgeted 4-0 Prolene suture on an RB needle. Transesophageal echocardiography did not identify any evidence of intracardiac gas.

Left ventricular venting was discontinued. The left ventricular vent catheter was removed, and the retaining pursestring suture was tied. The site was hemostatic without any requirement for repair sutures. Next, a test dose of protamine was administered, and continued until complete. During this time, decannulation was achieved. First, the inferior vena caval cannula was removed, and the retaining pursestring suture was tied. The site was hemostatic without any requirement for repair sutures. Next, the ascending thoracic aortic vent/antegrade cardioplegic catheter was removed, the retaining horizontal mattress suture was tied. The site was hemostatic without any requirement for repair sutures. Next, the superior vena caval cannula was removed, and both retaining pursestring sutures were tied. The site was hemostatic without any requirement for additional repair sutures. Finally, an appropriate systemic arterial blood pressure for ascending thoracic aortic decannulation was ensured/achieved. The ascending thoracic aortic cannula was removed, and the retaining pursestring sutures were tied. The site was hemostatic without any requirement for repair sutures. The quality of hemostasis in the mediastinum was satisfactory, but there was superficial with chest copious hemorrhage. The deep mediastinum and inclusive of the anastomotic and cannulation sites were packed with topical hemostatic agents (matrix cellulose/Nu-knit). The mediastinum was temporarily packed using meticulous pads.

Next, the AICD generator and leads were removed through a left lateral chest incision. This was performed without issue, and the incision was closed using layers of absorbable suture. Attention was once again focused in the mediastinum. The quality of hemostasis within the middle mediastinum, inclusive of all of the cannulation and anastomotic sites, was satisfactory. The aforementioned chest tubes were placed, exteriorized, and secured to the skin using 2-0 silk sutures.

There was severe hemorrhage from the sternum. Each hemi-sternum was repaired using heavy Vicryl suture in running fashion along the sternal edge. This appeared to improve hemostasis. Interlocking stainless steel sternal wires were placed to close the chest. The incision was closed using absorbable suture in layers, reinforced with interrupted nylon sutures of the skin. This concluded the case. Final sponge, needle, and instrument count were all correct. I was scrubbed and present for the entirety of the case.

Dr. Pham and I were co-surgeons for this case. I opened the patient, placed the patient on cardiopulmonary bypass, placed the vent and cardioplegia catheters, and performed the implantation of the donor cardiac allograft with the exception of the inferior vena caval anastomosis. Dr. Pham performed the native cardiectomy, left atrial appendage ligation, and the inferior vena caval anastomosis, which was quite challenging. This operation also took an extended period of time, due to the severe sternal bleeding. The actual cardiac transplantation procedure took approximately 4 hours and 30 minutes, while the process of achieving superficial mediastinal hemostasis at the level of the sternum and superficial soft tissues, took a total of 3 hours and 30 minutes.

ATTENDING PHYSICIANS STATEMENT: I was present for the entire procedure.

----[ Related Clinicians: Docnum#: 4116422 ]

PHAM, SI MAI ( CC )
RAJAGOPAL, KESHAVA ( DICT )
FELLER, ERIKA ( REFER )
RAJAGOPAL, KESHAVA ( SIGN 29-0CT-13)

End of Dictated Report

This document has been read and signed. Please contact the medical records department for any questions regarding this document.

END OF REPORT

APPENDIX

# Scripture Verses from Rev. David Drake

## Philippians 4:6-7
Be careful for nothing; but in every thing by prayer and supplication with thanksgiving let your requests be made known unto God. And the peace of God, which passeth all understanding, shall keep your hearts and minds through Christ Jesus.

## Philippians 1:6
And I am sure of this, that he who began a good work in you will bring it to completion at the day of Jesus Christ.

## Psalms 33:20-22
Our soul waits for the LORD; he is our help and our shield. For our heart is glad in him, because we trust in his holy name. Let your steadfast love, O LORD, be upon us, even as we hope in you.

## Jeremiah 29:11
For I know the plans I have for you, declares the LORD, plans for welfare and not for evil, to give you a future and a hope.

## Ecclesiastes 3:1
For everything there is a season, and a time for every matter under heaven.

## 2 Corinthians 1:3-4
Blessed be the God and Father of our Lord Jesus Christ, the Father of mercies and God of all comfort, who comforts us in all our affliction, so that we may be able to comfort those who are in any affliction, with the comfort with which we ourselves are comforted by God.

## 1 Peter 5:6-7
Humble yourselves, therefore, under the mighty hand of God so that at the proper time he may exalt you, casting all your anxieties on him, because he cares for you.

# About the Author

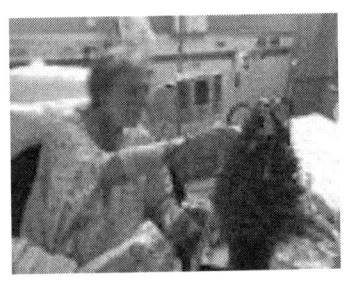

Vince Clews began his career as a scriptwriter, and eventually producer, for Maryland Public Television. He created and produced the popular PBS series *Consumer Survival Kit*. After Vince left public broadcasting, he spent the next several decades writing and producing video scripts for the clients of his production company, Vince Clews & Associates, Inc. His work has taken him around the world, including visits to many remote areas where he has seen firsthand the value of Non-Government Organizations in the lives of those who rely on the goodwill of givers and doers. We should be, at least, one or the other.

In 2013, Vince required—and by God's grace, received—a heart transplant. He continues to be in good health. Vince is the husband of Carol Clews. They each brought two children to their marriage. In order of age, they are Cristin, Chris, Todd, and Ashleigh. Vince and Carol have one grandchild, Kailey Rose Hitchcock.

Vince has a Bachelor's degree in English and Theater from Frostburg State University and an MS degree in Mass Communications from Indiana State University, Terre Haute, Indiana.

His first book is *Water Walkers: From Secular Careers to Sacred Service—39 Stories of Faith.*

Made in the USA
Middletown, DE
21 August 2020